Humanitarian Medicine and Disaster Relief

Focusing on emergency medical humanitarian assistance, this accessible new text provides practical clinical guidance for those working in emergency medicine, critical care, and military medicine. There has been great progress over the last 30 years in establishing standards and training programmes to ensure that those who respond to major emergencies are appropriately trained, adequately equipped, qualified to do this work, and accountable for the work that they do. These developments, together with insights into current requirements for healthcare and emergency responses, are reflected in this book.

The *Trauma Care Focus* series offers readers an opportunity to learn about specific aspects of trauma management in depth. The emphasis is on readability, and each book in the series will be short and informative rather than exhaustive. Each author is an acknowledged authority on their subject, with the content reflecting the most up-to-date knowledge.

Professor Tony Redmond is Professor Emeritus of International Emergency Medicine at the Humanitarian and Conflict Response Institute at the University of Manchester, and Emeritus Professor of Emergency Medicine at Keele University. He is the founder of UK-Med, the frontline medical aid charity, and served as its chairman for twenty-nine years until 2023. He was awarded an OBE in 1994 for his work providing humanitarian assistance in Sarajevo during the Bosnian war. Professor Redmond continues to work with the WHO, with whom he helped set up the Emergency Medical Teams Initiative, setting standards within the disaster relief field. He is a member of the executive committee of the Faculty of Remote Rural and Humanitarian Healthcare, based at the Royal College of Surgeons of Edinburgh.

Trauma Care Manuals and Trauma Care Focus
General Editor
Ian Greaves

Trauma Care Manuals
Trauma Care Manual 3rd Edition 2021
Trauma Care Pre-Hospital Manual 1st Edition 2019
(2nd Edition in preparation)
Trauma Care Manual of Trauma in Children (Due for
publication 2025)
Trauma Care Manual of Trauma in Women (In preparation)
Trauma Care Manual of War and Conflict Trauma
(In preparation)

Trauma Care Focus series
1. Humanitarian Medicine and Disaster Relief by Tony
   Redmond
2. Abdominal Trauma by Timothy Stansfield
3. Chemical, Biological, Radiation, and Nuclear Medicine by
   Steven Bland
4. Rehabilitation Medicine by John Etherington
5. Wound Care by Steven Jeffery

Humanitarian Medicine and Disaster Relief

Professor Tony Redmond OBE

Professor Emeritus of International Emergency Medicine
Humanitarian and Conflict Response Institute
University of Manchester

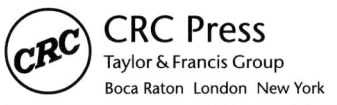

CRC Press
Taylor & Francis Group
Boca Raton London New York

CRC Press is an imprint of the
Taylor & Francis Group, an **informa** business

Designed series cover image: Shutterstock

First edition published 2025
by CRC Press
2385 NW Executive Center Drive, Suite 320, Boca Raton FL 33431

and by CRC Press
4 Park Square, Milton Park, Abingdon, Oxon, OX14 4RN

CRC Press is an imprint of Taylor & Francis Group, LLC

ISBN: 978-1-032-75377-5 (hbk)
ISBN: 978-1-032-75375-1 (pbk)
ISBN: 978-1-003-47371-8 (ebk)

DOI: 10.1201/9781003473718

Typeset in Minion
by Apex CoVantage, LLC

Dedication

I dedicate this book to all those humanitarian workers who give selflessly of themselves for the benefit of others while working in some of the most difficult and dangerous of circumstances, and from whom I have learned so much.

Contents

About the Author

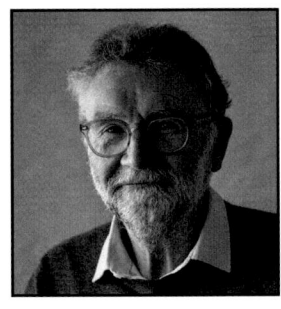 **Professor Tony Redmond** is the founder of UK-Med, the frontline medical aid charity, and served as its chairman for 29 years until 2023. During his time as chairman, UK-Med responded to requests for help from all corners of the world, most recently including Ukraine, and continues its work there whilst also running a range of programmes internationally, including Gaza, Lebanon, and Rwanda. Today, the organisation has more than 1000 highly trained UK and international doctors, nurses, paramedics and allied health professionals, aided by a central team of over 80. UK-Med provides experts, medical and surgical teams, and a full field hospital when required, to respond to outbreaks of infectious diseases, the consequences of chemical weapons, sudden-onset disasters, and conflicts, as well as running in-country healthcare programmes. Professor Redmond was awarded an OBE in 1994 for his work providing humanitarian assistance in Sarajevo during the Bosnian war, and the University of Manchester's Medal of Honour in 2018.

Professor Redmond, who grew up in Failsworth and originally studied medicine at the University of Manchester, is a consultant in emergency medicine, professor emeritus of international emergency medicine at the Humanitarian and Conflict Response

Institute at the University of Manchester, emeritus professor of emergency medicine at Keele University, and past president of the World Association for Disaster and Emergency Medicine.

Although he has stood down from an executive role with UK-Med, Professor Redmond remains its official ambassador and continues to work with the WHO, with whom he helped set up the Emergency Medical Teams Initiative, setting standards within the disaster relief field. He is a member of the executive committee of the Faculty of Remote Rural and Humanitarian Healthcare at the Royal College of Surgeons of Edinburgh.

Professor Redmond is the author of *Frontline: Saving Lives in War, Disaster and Disease* (HarperNorth 2021).

Editor's Introduction

The series of *Trauma Care Manuals*, which continues to expand, offers evidence-based guidelines for the management of trauma victims, and the first two manuals are now established as standard trauma texts. This new series of publications, *Trauma Care Focus*, of which this is the first, offers readers an opportunity to learn about specific aspects of trauma management to a greater depth than is possible in the manuals. The emphasis, however, will be on readability. Each book in the series will be short, informative, and entertaining rather than exhaustive, but characterised by having been written by an acknowledged authority on the subject and reflecting up-to-date knowledge.

This first *Focus* sets a very high standard. We are honoured that Prof Tony Redmond has written it for us and delighted that he has been willing to share his unsurpassed experience and wisdom. We hope you enjoy it and find it useful.

Ian Greaves
2024

Preface

When medical care on a huge scale is needed, it is commonly supposed that '*any help is better than no help*'. However, medical assistance, even in the most extreme of circumstances, requires skill and training. Primum non nocere, or "*first do no harm*", has been central to the concept of good medical practice since the time of Hippocrates: "*I will use treatment to help the sick according to my ability and judgment, but never with a view to injury and wrong-doing*." Implicit in this commitment is that a good physician, or indeed any other healthcare worker, will practice only within their field of proven competence. Just as we recognise that emergency departments are no longer places where those in need of training go to gain experience from those in need of care, but rather must be places where those in need of care go to gain from the experience of experts, this approach must be extended to the management of large-scale disasters and international humanitarian emergencies. There has been great progress over the last 30 years in establishing standards and training programmes to ensure that those who respond to major emergencies are appropriately trained, adequately equipped, qualified to do this work, and accountable for the work that they do. These developments will be described, along with the milestones on the way to their establishment.

Tony Redmond

(Please Note - Each chapter can be read independently and therefore key messages are sometimes repeated).

Abbreviations

CBRN	Chemical Biological Radiation and Nuclear
CMR	Crude Mortality Rate
COPD	Chronic Obstructive Pulmonary Disease
CT	Computerised Tomography
EmOC	Emergency Obstetric Care
EMT	Emergency Medical Team
EMTCC	Emergency Medical Team Coordination Cell
ERC	Emergency Relief Coordinator
GDP	Gross Domestic Product
GOARN	Global Outbreak Alert and Response Network
HEAT	Hostile Environment Awareness Training
IASC	Inter-Agency Standing Committee
ICRC	International Committee of the Red Cross
IDP	Internally Displaced Person
IFRC	International Federation of Red Cross and Red Crescent Societies
IHL	International Humanitarian Law
INSARAG	International Search and Rescue Advisory Group
IPC	Infection Prevention and Control
IRS	Indoor Residual Spraying
ISAR	International Search and Rescue
LLIN	Long-Lasting Insecticidal Net
MESS	Mangled Extremity Severity Score
MoH	Ministry of Health
MSF	Medicines San Frontières

MUAC	Middle Upper Arm Circumference
NGO	Non-Governmental Organisation
OCHA	(United Nations) Office for the Coordination of Humanitarian Affairs
ORS	Oral Rehydration Salts
OSOCC	On-Site Operations Coordination Centre
OXFAM	Oxford Committee for Famine Relief
PAHO	Pan-American Health Organisation
PEP	Post Exposure Prophylaxis
PFA	Psychological First Aid
PPE	Personal Protection Equipment
SCF	Save the Children Fund
SGBV	Sexual and Gender-Based Violence
STI	Sexually Transmitted Infection
TTD	Transfusion Transmittable Disease
UN	United Nations (Organisation)
UNDAC	United Nations Disaster Assessment and Coordination Team
UNDRR	United Nations Office for Disaster Risk Reduction
UNHCR	United Nations High Commissioner for Refugees
USAR	Urban Search and Rescue
VOSOCC	Virtual On-Site Operations Coordination Centre
WASH	Water Sanitation and Hygiene
WCDRR	World Conference on Disaster Risk Reduction
WHOCC	World Health Organisation Coordination Center

Illustration Credits

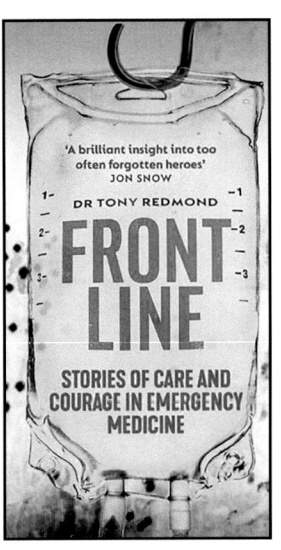

Figures 8.2 and 10.1 are from Wikimedia Commons and used under the Creative Commons License. Table 3.1 is adapted from Wikimedia Commons. Figure 3.3 is in the public domain. All other illustrations were provided by the author or are copyright Trauma Care and used with permission.

1

Humanitarianism

It is important at the outset to agree on what we understand by the words *humanitarian* and *humanitarianism*. In everyday conversation, when we describe a person or an act as "humanitarian", we generally mean that the person or their actions and intentions are good and that they are acting for the overall benefit of mankind or at least a portion of it. Humanitarianism, therefore, has similarities in this context to the concept of altruism. The concept of humanitarianism, certainly in the West, arose particularly in the mid-to-late 19th century when it was linked to the word 'humane', and associated with the many social reforms that were then taking place. Of particular importance in the genesis of humanitarianism was the work of Henri Dunant, who founded the International Committee of the Red Cross (ICRC) in 1863 and was instrumental in the establishment of the Geneva Conventions. It was the suffering and neglect of the wounded in battle that inspired Dunant to write his seminal work, *A Memory of Solferino,* and shortly afterwards to galvanise the formation of the ICRC in Geneva as an independent organisation that advocated for the better treatment of those wounded in war. He also advocated for the establishment of national groups of volunteers to assist the wounded in times of conflict.[1] One year after the ICRC was founded, the first *Geneva Convention* was drawn up and agreed. This treaty obliged armies to care for wounded soldiers, whichever side they were on, and the Red Cross emblem for medical services was introduced.

DOI: 10.1201/9781003473718-1

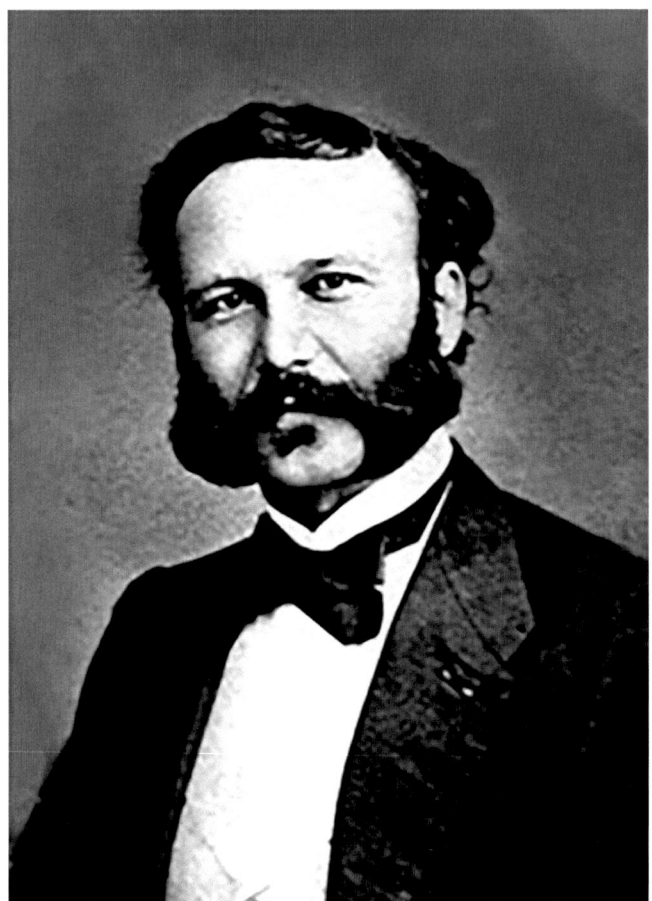

Figure 1.1 Henri Dunant

The choice of a red cross on a white background was chosen as the reversal of the Swiss flag. During the First World War, the ICRC opened the Central Prisoners of War Agency in Geneva, to restore links between captured soldiers and their families. The Great War also saw a mass mobilisation of national societies to look after the wounded. Shortly after the Second World War, in 1949, the now three Geneva Conventions, covering the wounded and sick on the battlefield, victims of war at sea, and prisoners of war, were revised and a fourth convention to protect civilians living under enemy control[2] was added, along with a number of additional protocols.[3]

Now, whenever there is a need for international assistance the term used to describe it is a *humanitarian emergency,* and the corresponding assistance is *humanitarian aid.* However, it is important to understand that the term *humanitarian* in these circumstances has a specific meaning. It requires that those involved, and their actions, adhere to the *humanitarian principles.* These principles are summarised as follows:

- Humanity
- Neutrality
- Impartiality
- Independence

> **Humanity.** Human suffering must be addressed wherever it is found. The purpose of humanitarian action is to protect life and health and ensure respect for human beings.
> **Neutrality.** Humanitarian actors must not take sides in hostilities or engage in controversies of a political, racial, religious, or ideological nature.
> **Impartiality.** Humanitarian action must be carried out on the basis of need alone, giving priority to the most urgent cases of distress and making no distinctions on the basis of nationality, race, gender, religion, class, or political opinions.
> **Independence.** Humanitarian action must be autonomous and independent of the political, economic, military, or other objectives that any actor may hold with regard to areas where humanitarian action is being implemented.

In 1997, a number of humanitarian agencies, including the ICRC, established the Humanitarian Charter. Within the charter is the recognition of the rights and duties laid down in international law. At the heart of these lie three fundamental rights:

- the right to live with dignity,
- the right to receive humanitarian assistance,
- the right to protection and security.

The charter also requires, firstly, that when delivering aid, the humanitarian imperative comes first, and that aid is given regardless of the race, creed, or nationality of the recipients, and without adverse distinction of any kind. Secondly, that aid priorities will be calculated on the basis of need alone and will not be used to further a particular political or religious standpoint, and thirdly, that those wishing to be seen as humanitarians shall endeavour not to act as instruments of government foreign policy and shall respect local cultures and customs.

At the same time these agencies identified a set of humanitarian standards to be applied in all humanitarian responses—the Sphere Standards.[4] These are grouped into four sections—

- water supply, sanitation, and hygiene promotion (WASH)
- food security and nutrition
- shelter and settlement
- health

These fundamentals of humanitarianism are applicable to all organisations, whether they are government organisations, non-government organisations (NGOs), the Red Cross/Red Crescent Societies, the ICRC, or the UN. They combine with the Geneva Conventions, the later Hague Conventions, and other legal frameworks into the concept of International Humanitarian Law (IHL).[5]

IHL is *"a set of rules that seeks, for humanitarian reasons, to limit the effects of armed conflict"*. It protects those who are not, or are no longer, directly or actively participating in hostilities, and imposes limits on the means and methods of warfare. An important component of IHL is the concept of *hors de combat*. Once wounded, taken prisoner, or having surrendered, these individuals, now non-combatants, are protected and are to be given the same care, including medical care, as civilians or one's own wounded combatants.

Following on from the establishment of the ICRC in Geneva, there are now many humanitarian organisations around the world. National Red Cross or Red Crescent organisations are present in many countries and come together under the International

Federation of the Red Cross/Red Crescent Societies (IFRC), also situated in Geneva, alongside its sister organisation, the ICRC. Those humanitarian organisations not part of the ICRC/IFRC or the UN are usually referred to as "Non-Government Organisations", or NGOs. One of the most successful is Medicines San Frontières (Doctors without Borders), known usually as MSF.

Many NGOs have their origins in war. MSF, for example, was founded in France in 1971 by a group of doctors and journalists in the wake of war and famine in Biafra, Nigeria. Some of the founders had worked for the ICRC, and their aim was to establish an organisation that focused on delivering emergency medical aid quickly, effectively, impartially, and independently.[6] The Save the Children Fund, or SCF as it is known now, was founded in the UK in 1919 by Eglantyne Jebb and Dorothy Buxton to alleviate starvation amongst the populations of Germany and its allies immediately after the First World War. In 1942, the Oxford Committee for Famine Relief (officially shortened to OXFAM in 1962) was established to support the starving in war-torn Greece during WWII.

Other NGOs are faith-based. For example, World Vision was founded in 1950 as an Ecumenical Christian organisation, and Islamic Relief was established in the UK in 1984.

While humanitarian action can be linked to religious belief and/or religious organisations, to be considered a humanitarian organisation, the humanitarian principles must still be upheld, and aid distributed according to need and not religion.

Governments may respond to humanitarian crises, including by dispatching emergency medical teams, but if their interventions are to be considered humanitarian, they too must adhere to all the humanitarian principles, including allowing their teams to distribute aid impartially, neutrally, and independently.

Compliance with all the humanitarian principles is most likely to be threatened when humanitarian organisations look to work *alongside* or occasionally *with* the military, when neutrality, impartiality, and independence might be, or appear to be, compromised. The United Nations Office for the Coordination of Humanitarian Affairs (OCHA) has published *Guidelines on the Use of Foreign Military and Civil Defence Assets in Disaster Relief,* the *Oslo Guidelines*.[7] A core principle of these is that use of the military must only be as a last resort.

It becomes even more difficult to maintain the humanitarian principles when humanitarian organisations are required to embed within the military during a conflict. For example, in Mosul in 2017, the Iraqi government had insisted on emergency medical teams being embedded with the Iraqi army, a condition too far away from the humanitarian principles for many organisations, which meant they could not respond despite the obvious need. The WHO, in its role as the *agent of last resort*, directly recruited and employed a range of organisations who were willing to deploy. Such was the international concern within the humanitarian community about this response that the WHO commissioned Johns Hopkins University to produce a report.[8] They found that the WHO and its partners had emphasised the first humanitarian principle, the imperative to save lives, above other humanitarian principles such as independence, neutrality, and, some claimed, impartiality. They concluded that "medical teams working directly with a combatant force should not be identified as humanitarian groups".

One final point to make about the word "humanitarian" is that it is also used in practice as a shorthand for emergency aid, to distinguish it from long-term development aid. But even when used in this context, the principles outlined here still apply.

MIGRATION

Much international humanitarian effort is aimed at people on the move, and it is important to understand the various labels and status of the different groups. *Refugees* are people who have fled war, violence, conflict, or persecution, and have *crossed an international border* to find safety in another country. *IDPs (internally displaced persons)* have been forced to flee their homes for similar reasons as refugees, but *have not crossed an international border* and still live in their countries of origin. *Asylum-seekers* are people who have fled their homes and claim international protection, but whose status has not yet been definitively determined. Every refugee begins as an asylum-seeker, but not every asylum-seeker will be granted refugee status. **Migrants** are people who move between temporary homes, either within their home country or internationally. This is different from an immigrant, who makes the conscious decision to move and resettle in a new country.

CLIMATE CHANGE, CONFLICT, AND HUMAN DISPLACEMENT [9]

The threat of violence is not the only reason for forced migration. Lack of work due to a combination of factors, including conflict and agricultural degradation, will force people to move on from their country of origin.[10]

Increasing numbers of people are fleeing persecution, violence, and human rights violations caused or exacerbated by the social impacts of climate change and the agricultural and weather-related disasters that follow. When families move in large numbers, they can place considerable strain on local health services, particularly primary care.[11]

The office of the United Nations High Commissioner for Refugees, UNHCR, is mandated by the United Nations to protect and safeguard the rights of refugees, former refugees who have returned to their home country, people displaced within their own country, and people who are stateless or whose nationality is disputed. It is guided by, and acts as the guardian of, the 1951 Refugee Convention[12] and its 1967 Protocol. The core principle of the 1951 Convention is *non-refoulement*, which asserts that a refugee should not be returned to a country where they face serious threats to their life or freedom. The document outlines the basic minimum standards for the treatment of refugees, including the right to housing, work, and education while displaced so they can lead a dignified and independent life. It also defines a refugee's obligations to the host country and specifies certain categories of people, such as war criminals, who do not qualify for refugee status. In addition, it details the legal obligations of the states that are party to one or both of these instruments.

NOTES AND REFERENCES

1. His book is available to download free of charge from the ICRC website. https://www.icrc.org/en/publication/0361-memory-solferino
2. https://www.icrc.org/
3. https://ihl-databases.icrc.org/
4. https://www.spherestandards.org/handbook
5. https://www.icrc.org/en/law-and-policy
6. https://www.msf.org/who-we-are
7. https://www.unocha.org/publications/report/world/oslo-guidelines-guidelines-use-foreign-military-and-civil-defence-assets-disaster-relief-revision-11-november-
8. Spiegel, P. B., Garber, K., Kushner, A., and Wise, P. The Mosul Trauma Response. A Case Study. The Johns Hopkins Center for Humanitarian Research; 2018 February.
9. https://www.unhcr.org/uk/what-we-do/build-better-futures/environment-disasters-and-climate-change/climate-change-and
10. https://www.concern.org.uk/news/refugee-migrant-idp-whats-difference?gclid
11. https://www.uk-med.org/ukraine
12. https://www.unhcr.org/uk/about-unhcr/who-we-are/1951-refugee-convention

2

Sudden-Onset Disasters

According to the UN, a disaster occurs when there is a serious disruption of the functioning of a community or a society at any scale due to hazardous events interacting with conditions of exposure, vulnerability, and capacity, leading to one or more of the following: human, material, economic, and environmental losses and impacts.[1]

Disasters have been commonly divided into *natural* and *man-made*, but such distinctions are generally artificial. All disasters are to a greater or lesser extent human-made, and are a function of where and how people choose or, in particular, are forced to live. The trigger may be a natural phenomenon such as an earthquake, but its impact will be determined by the prior vulnerability of the affected community. Poverty is the single most important factor in determining vulnerability: poor countries have weak infrastructure, and poor people cannot afford to move to safer places. Whatever the disaster, an additional threat to health often comes from the mass movement of people away from the scene and into inadequate temporary facilities.

Despite this, and although this distinction is used less widely than previously, it is still to some extent customary to divide disasters into natural and man-made. However, by using the word "natural" there is an implication that the disaster and/or its consequences are inevitable; an "act of God". The use of the term *accident* has largely been abandoned in medical parlance in the UK,[2] as it is accepted that these events are not unpredictable, rarely inevitable, and almost always preventable or capable of mitigation. The same is true of disasters. There are obviously *natural phenomena* that create

DOI: 10.1201/9781003473718-2   9

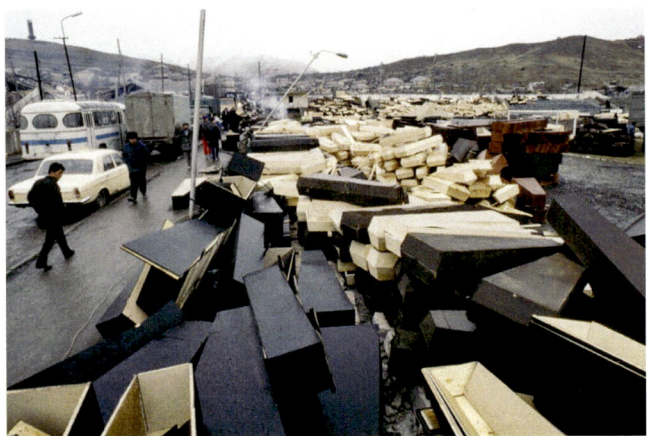

Figure 2.1 A scene from the Armenian Earthquake 1988

natural hazards for populations when they occur, but the disaster that potentially follows is not always inevitable, and to a greater or lesser degree is man-made—due to a lack of planning, lack of preparation, or an inadequate response.[3] By way of example, the first large-scale international response to a major "natural" disaster was in 1988 following a 6.8 magnitude earthquake in Armenia, where tens of thousands of people perished (Figure 2.1).

The following year, in 1989, a stronger earthquake of 6.9 magnitude struck the Loma Prieta area of California, and 67 people died. These were both natural phenomena, but the disaster that followed each was not natural, nor was it inevitable. It was determined by the quality of the buildings that were affected. In turn, the quality of the buildings was determined by the financial and political capacity of the state where they were built. The poor are always the most vulnerable to disasters, and the very poorest in the world the most vulnerable of all. But poverty too is not inevitable; it is a product of the politics and economics that govern not only architecture, but also disaster planning, preparedness, and response.

While disasters are increasing in frequency across the world (Figure 2.2),[4] their death toll has decreased remarkably over the last hundred years or so (Figure 2.3).[5] However, the deaths that

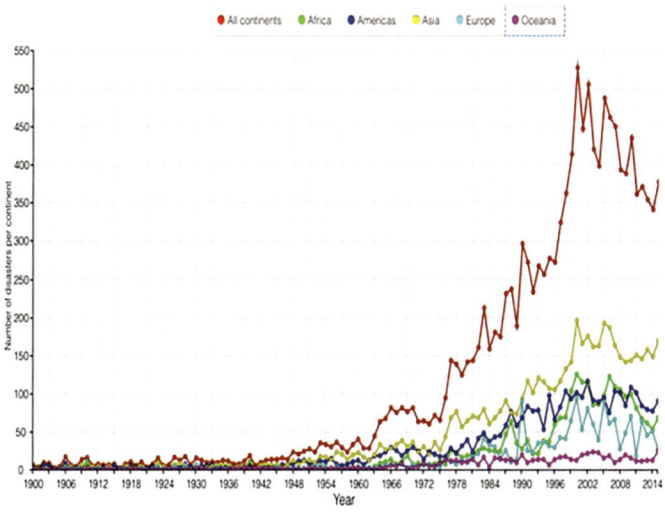

Figure 2.2 Total number of reported natural disasters between 1900 and 2015

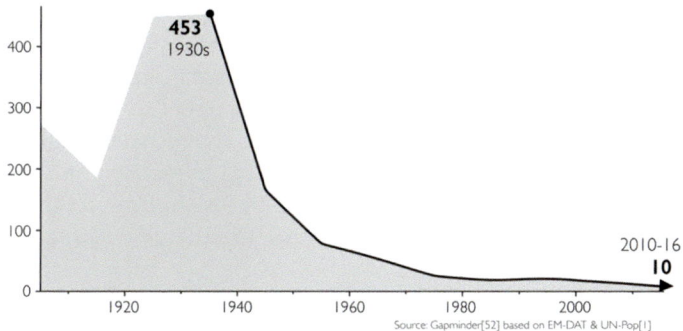

Figure 2.3 Deaths from disaster: annual deaths per million people, 10 year averages

arise from these disasters are now concentrated among the poorest people living in the poorest countries.

Those from poorer economic backgrounds in fact bear over two-thirds of the world trauma burden, irrespective of disasters, with far higher rates of death from injury and with more non-fatal injuries than in higher-income countries. People with life-threatening but survivable injuries are also six times more likely to die in a low-income setting (36% mortality) than in a high-income setting (6% mortality),[6] irrespective of an intervening disaster.

When considering the impact of a disaster, it is essential to include its total effect, including economic, human, and environmental consequences. These will include deaths, injuries, disease, and negative effects on human physical, mental, and social well-being. The annual losses caused by earthquakes, tsunamis, cyclones, winds, and tidal waves are estimated to represent between 1.2% and 1.7% of the world's gross domestic product (GDP).[7] As described here, it is not solely the fact that these events have occurred that indicates a concomitant disaster, but whether the event and its consequences are *uncompensated*. An uncompensated major incident is one where the medical and other responding services are destroyed or rendered totally inadequate.

In terms of the impact of a disaster on health systems, it is imperative to understand that not only is there an obvious direct impact consequent upon the nature of the event; for example, many patients after an earthquake requiring treatment for injuries or infected patients in a disease outbreak, but there is also an indirect impact on patients with coincidental emergencies and chronic conditions who will continue to present to what are now overwhelmed health facilities. Obstetric emergencies, victims of road traffic collisions, and those suffering myocardial infarction or acute abdominal pain will now be treated in facilities that are depleted, damaged, or may even have been largely destroyed by the disaster.

In addition, those with long-term or chronic conditions may find their ongoing needs severely, or even completely, compromised. These secondary effects are likely to particularly affect those countries with an already vulnerable healthcare system which may have only just been managing to meet the chronic health needs of the population before the disaster occurred. If these issues are not adequately addressed, deaths and disability from these secondary consequences may end up outnumbering those from the immediate, direct consequences of the disaster.

Disasters can have a long tail. The disruption to a health system may last months, and in already vulnerable countries, sometimes years. Although international teams can often arrive too late to perform immediate life-saving surgery, they can support the maintenance and re-establishment of the health services, and carry out much-needed reconstructive surgery and rehabilitation in the severely injured patients who need it.[8]

DISASTER RISK REDUCTION

The United Nations Office for Disaster Risk Reduction (UNDRR) has published the *Sendai Framework* for disaster risk reduction.[9] The priorities for action are identified as:

- understanding disaster risk
- strengthening disaster risk governance to manage disaster risk
- investing in disaster risk reduction for resilience
- enhancing disaster preparedness for effective response and to *build back better* in recovery, rehabilitation, and reconstruction

This framework was endorsed by the UN General Assembly following the 2015 Third UN World Conference on Disaster Risk Reduction (WCDRR), and advocates "the substantial reduction of disaster risk and losses in lives, livelihoods and health and in the economic, physical, social, cultural and environmental assets of persons, businesses, communities and countries". It is the successor to the Hyogo Framework for Action (HFA) 2005–2015.[10]

Within the Sendai framework is the following useful terminology:

- **small-scale disaster**: a type of disaster only affecting local communities which require assistance beyond the affected community.

- **large-scale disaster**: a type of disaster affecting a society which requires national or international assistance.
- **frequent and infrequent disasters**: this distinction depends on the probability of occurrence and the return period of a given hazard and its impacts. The impact of frequent disasters can be cumulative or become chronic for a community or a society.
- A **slow-onset disaster** is defined as one that emerges gradually over time. Slow-onset disasters could be associated with, for example, drought, desertification, sea-level rise, or epidemic disease outbreak.
- A **sudden-onset disaster** is one triggered by a hazardous event that emerges quickly or unexpectedly. Sudden-onset disasters might be associated with, for example, an earthquake, volcanic eruption, flash flood, chemical explosion, critical infrastructure failure, or transport accident.

The Sendai framework has a number of targets, including substantially reducing global disaster mortality by 2030 (aiming to lower the average per hundred thousand global mortality between 2020–2030 compared to 2005–2015), as well as the number of affected people globally by 2030, aiming to lower the average global figure per hundred thousand over the same time period. The framework also sets a target of reducing the economic effects directly due to disasters in relation to global GDP and reducing disaster damage to critical infrastructure and disruption of basic services, among them health and educational facilities, including through developing their resilience, by 2030. Targets to increase the number of countries with national and local disaster risk reduction strategies by 2020 and to enhance international cooperation with developing countries through adequate and sustainable support to complement their national actions for implementation of this framework by 2030 were also set, as was an aspiration to increase the availability of, and access to, multi-hazard early warning systems and disaster risk information and assessments by 2030.

NOTES AND REFERENCES

1. https://www.undrr.org
2. Accidents are not unpredictable, Davis, R. M., North American, editor, and Barry Pless, editor. Injury Prevention. *BMJ*. 2001 June 2; 322 (7298): 1320–1321.
3. https://www.undrr.org/our-impact/campaigns/no-natural-disasters
4. Catholic University of Louvain in Brussels runs the CRED International Disaster Database—EMDAT Centre for Research on the epidemiology of disasters
5. https://www.gapminder.org
6. https://www.who.int/initiatives/global-alliance-for-care-of-the-injured
7. https://www.paho.org/en/health-emergencies/disaster-risk-reduction
8. https://isprm.org/
9. https://www.undrr.org/implementing-sendai-framework/what-sendai-framework
10. https://www.unisdr.org/2005/wcdr/intergover/official-doc/L-docs/Hyogo-framework-for-action-english.pdf

3

Specific Hazards

EARTHQUAKES

Earthquake tremors occur with the movement of the earth's crust along tectonic plates. Such tremors occur every day, often large ones, with most, fortunately, occurring out at sea and posing little or no threat to human populations.

The point nearest to the surface is called the epicentre (epi being Greek for 'above') and the site where the force of the earthquake is felt the strongest (Figure 3.1). The force of an earthquake is measured on the Richter Scale. This is a logarithmic, not linear, scale, rising in multiples of 10, so a force 7 quake, for example, is 10 times stronger than a force 6 and 100 times stronger than a force 5 (Table 3.1).

It is a truism that earthquakes have never killed anyone. It is falling buildings that kill people, crushing or trapping occupants or injuring those nearby with debris. High-income countries can afford to build stronger, earthquake-resistant buildings, but poorer countries are inevitably worse affected by earthquakes of similar magnitude.

In terms of search and rescue, the floors of poorly constructed multistorey buildings may collapse onto each other, leaving little chance of survival for the occupants. However, floors may partially collapse and create cavities in which minimally injured occupants may survive, at least for a short time. Earthquakes at night when occupants are at home are deadlier in residential properties, and

 DOI: 10.1201/9781003473718-3

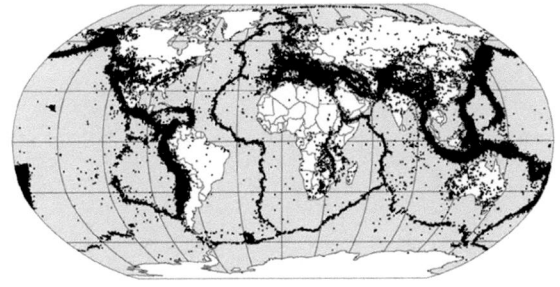

Figure 3.1 Distribution of earthquake epicentres 1963–1998

schools more vulnerable in the day when children are in class. Survival during entrapment is obviously dependent on the severity of any injuries that have been incurred, but also on the availability of oxygen and water. Food is not an absolute requirement, at least for several weeks, as long as adequate water is available.

When considering International Search and Rescue (ISAR), it is important to appreciate that most survivors will be rescued by fellow victims. They are the nearest at hand, and most successful rescues will take place within the first 24 hours. They will be joined by local, and then national, rescue teams. When needed, additional specialist teams can be called upon to search for those deeply entrapped, including international search and rescue teams. However, because of the time it may take for these teams to arrive on scene, the rescue rate may be low.

It is important, therefore, that high-income and well-resourced countries look to strengthen the local and regional search and rescue capacity in earthquake-prone countries. This is an area where the experience and resources of high-income countries can be used to good effect in working with and supporting teams in low- and middle-income countries.

The International Search and Rescue Advisory Group (INSARAG)[1] at the UN has a classification and verification system to establish and maintain standards for search and rescue teams, and it publishes its guidelines.[2]

It is the nature of earthquakes that in urban areas with building collapse and falling debris, up to three times as many people

Table 3.1 The Richter Scale

Magnitude	Description	EMS-98*	What it feels like	Frequency
1.0–1.9	Micro	I	Not felt.	Continual
2.0–2.9	Minor	I	Felt slightly by some people. No damage to buildings.	> one million per year
3.0–3.9	Slight	II to III	Often felt by people, very rarely causes damage.	>100,000 per year
4.0–4.9	Light	IV to V	Felt by most people in the affected area. Usually zero to minimal damage.	10,000–15,000 per year
5.0–5.9	Moderate	VI to VII	Can cause damage of varying severity to poorly constructed buildings.	1,000–1,500 per year
6.0–6.9	Strong	VII to IX	Damage to a moderate number of well-built structures in populated areas. Earthquake-resistant structures survive with slight to moderate damage. Strong to violent shaking in the epicentral area.	100–150 per year
7.0–7.9	Major	VIII or higher	Causes damage to most buildings. Well-designed structures are likely to receive damage. Major damage mostly limited to 250 km from the epicenter.	10–20 per year
8.0–8.9	Great		Major damage to buildings, moderate to heavy damage to sturdy or earthquake-resistant buildings. Damage over large areas. Felt over very large areas.	One per year
9.0–9.9	Extreme		Near total destruction. Permanent changes in ground topography.	One to three per century

*European Macroseismic Scale. https://www.gfz.de/en/section/seismic-hazard-and-risk-dynamics/data-products-services/ems-98-european-macroseismic-scale are injured as are killed. The pressure on local hospital facilities can therefore be enormous. Major head and chest injuries are rapidly fatal, and intra-abdominal bleeding will require immediate intervention by on-site surgeons if survival is to be secured. This means that incoming surgeons from other countries will inevitably arrive too late to carry out immediately lifesaving surgery. However, many of the survivors will have incurred peripheral limb injuries, which represent the commonest longer-term surgical problems after a large-scale earthquake. Prolonged compression produces crush injuries. These require early surgical intervention to restore circulation and prevent infection and thereby allow the possibility of limb salvage. Crush injuries with associated fluid loss and rhabdomyolysis can lead to the development of crush syndrome and renal failure. It is imperative therefore that appropriate resuscitation and surgery are carried out as soon as possible to prevent this. This is where incoming surgical teams can provide a much-needed surge in capacity for the local health services. "Orthoplastics" is therefore an essential component of emergency medical teams responding to large-scale earthquakes.

The greatest impacts of earthquakes will often be non-medical, with the loss of communications, transport, and power disrupting all aspects of daily life, including the provision of healthcare.

There is a natural, but in fact unfounded, fear of the unburied dead causing disease and epidemics.[3] This can be amplified after earthquakes, when there may be hundreds, even thousands, of dead bodies lying unburied in public places. It has been well established that sudden-onset disasters do not of themselves precipitate epidemics. It is the mass movement of people into inadequate temporary accommodations, with their associated poor water quality and hygiene facilities, that can lead to increased cases of diarrhoeal disease and facilitate the spread of respiratory infections. However, the unburied dead themselves pose little or no threat to the living in these circumstances. It is the living who are the threat when there are inadequate WASH facilities. If, on the other hand, death has occurred as the result of an infection that remains infectious after the death of its host (in practice principally cholera and viral haemorrhagic fevers such as Ebola), then those handling dead bodies may become infected and so spread disease.

TSUNAMI (TIDAL WAVE)

A tsunami occurs when a seismic eruption at sea triggers a powerful wave of water which is slowed as it approaches land by the rising shoreline, and it transfers the energy of its horizontal movement upwards into a wall of water. Buildings are destroyed both by the initial impact of this moving mass of water, as well as by the drag of the receding sea pulling on foundations and eroding the ground beneath. In addition, debris is gathered in the moving water, adding further to its destructive effect.

Whereas in earthquakes there may be three injured for every death, it is essentially the reverse in a tsunami, when deaths, usually from drowning, can outnumber the injured by as much is 9:1 (Figure 3.2). It is an unavoidable fact that the severely injured are unlikely to be able to swim, so survivors are likely to have either avoided the tsunami altogether by moving to higher ground, or to have suffered only relatively minor injuries. This has implications for emergency medical assistance. The need for international surgical teams will be limited, but the destruction of essential healthcare services will often require a broader range of support to re-establish and maintain health care to the affected population.

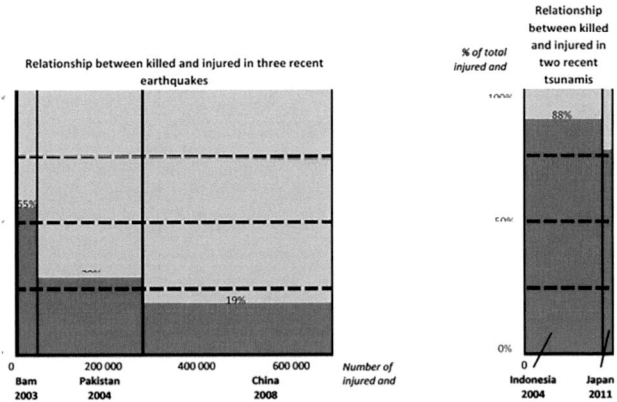

Figure 3.2 Mortality (dark gray) and morbidity (light gray) ratios for earthquakes and tsunamis compared.

Source: CRED EM-DAT

The greatest need for assistance is usually for help in road clearance and rebuilding. Rebuilding is often best carried out by local and national authorities, and where outside help is required, this is usually requested in the form of financial assistance.

LANDSLIDES

Persistent heavy rain can destabilise hillsides, particularly in areas of deforestation (a human-made rather than natural phenomenon) (Figure 3.3). Mudflows can also follow tsunamis, floods in

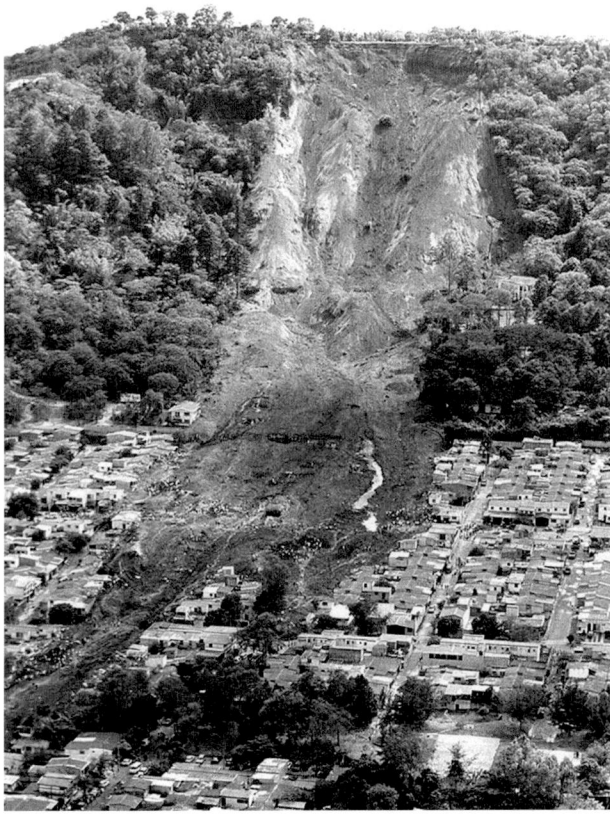

Figure 3.3 A landslide in El Salvador

general, and occasionally earthquakes affecting vulnerable land. Those trapped in the mud will be subjected to the compressive forces of the mud, which over time will produce crush injuries and ultimately crush syndrome. Intravenous fluid loading before, during, and after rescue may protect against a catastrophic fall in blood pressure that can follow the sudden release of compressed tissues after prolonged entrapment. This phenomenon must also be factored into the rescue of those trapped in fallen buildings from any cause where there has been a prolonged period of tissue compression.

FLOODS

Severe flooding will obviously lead to deaths from drowning, including the deaths of those trapped in cars, especially in fast-flowing water. In addition, damage to crops and infrastructure can have a profound effect on life in general, as well as the ability to provide healthcare in particular. Water supplies may also be at risk of contamination with sewage, leading to an increased risk of diarrhoeal disease.

VOLCANIC ERUPTIONS

Because volcanic ash eventually provides highly fertile soil, areas vulnerable to volcanic activity are often surprisingly well-populated. When a volcano erupts, more injuries in survivors are likely to have occurred in those rushing to escape, or from falling rocks and debris, than from burns. However, people do incur severe burn injuries in lava flows, although these are often fatal. Pyroclastic flows of lava (horizontal blasts of gas containing ash and larger fragments in suspension) move very quickly, destroying and igniting everything, and everyone, in their path.

Ash-falls will produce respiratory injuries and inhalational burns. In practice, only those whose burns are superficial and to the upper airways will survive. Exposure to volcanic ash will provoke excessive mucus production and the formation of mucus plugs, leading to acute respiratory distress as well as exacerbations of asthma. There is a theoretical concern about the risk of silicosis

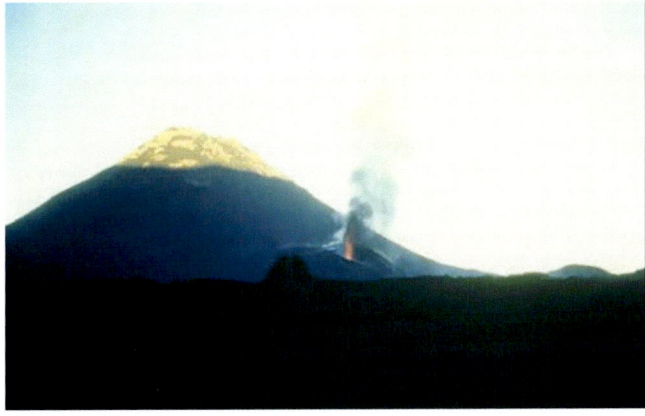

Figure 3.4 A volcanic eruption in Cape Verde. The eruption Itself caused few deaths or injuries, but a cholera outbreak followed the mass evacuation of local people to tented accommodation in a neighbouring island where cholera was already endemic.

from inhalation of silica particles, but in practice the exposure will usually have been too short-lived for this to be significant. Nevertheless, other toxic gases may be emitted, and poisoning from carbon monoxide, hydrofluoric acid, and sulphur dioxide can occur.

As in all sudden-onset disasters, it is the destruction of facilities that produces the most lasting damage, and the loss of health facilities in particular poses the biggest threat to wellbeing (Figure 3.4).

TROPICAL STORMS

International convention dictates that tropical storms in the Indian Ocean are called cyclones, those in the North Atlantic, Caribbean, and South Pacific, are called hurricanes, and those in the North and West Pacific, are called typhoons. They are the result of humid air rising upwards from warm sea water into cooler air above. Over the sea, the air can move at speeds of more than 300 kph. They can be extremely destructive, with flying debris causing severe injuries. The associated heavy rainfall can also lead to significant flooding.

When Typhoon Tracy struck the town of Darwin in the Northern Territories of Australia in 1974, many of the roofs were made of corrugated iron that had been secured to the rafters with metal bolts. These proved insufficient to withstand wind gusts of over 200 km/h, and sheets of corrugated iron and bolts became airborne missiles that wreaked havoc on the population of the town. Since then, very strict building regulations have ensured that buildings are strong and able to withstand such high winds, providing a good example of how the disasters that follow natural phenomena can, and should, be mitigated.

FAMINE

Disasters and conflicts can precipitate acute food shortages, particularly where there is socioeconomic and political instability. Recognised trigger levels for urgent humanitarian intervention include a rise in crude mortality to 1 in 10,000 a day, pronounced wasting in individuals (loss of >15% of normal body weight), and food energy supplies of <1500 kcal a day. Famines both cause humanitarian crises and occur as a result of them. They can often precipitate the mass movement of people, further compounding the precipitating emergency.

NOTES AND REFERENCES

1. https://www.insarag.org/
2. https://www.insarag.org/methodology/insarag-guidelines/
3. PAHO/WHO. Management of Dead Bodies after Disasters: A Field Manual for First Responders. 2nd edition (Revised). PAHO/WHO (Pan American Health Organization); 2018. https://www.paho.org/en/documents/management-dead-bodies-after-disasters-field-manual-first-responders-2nd-edition-revised

4

Responding to Humanitarian Emergencies

A humanitarian emergency *is an event, or series of events, that represents a critical threat to the health, safety, security or wellbeing of a community or other large group of people, usually over a wide area.*[1] The need for medical assistance in such humanitarian emergencies, and disasters in general, continues to rise. The UN emphasises too that humanitarian emergencies created by conflicts are widespread and protracted, with significant injuries to the civilian population. However, where those providing medical care to the ill and injured in war might once have expected a degree of protection, attacks on healthcare[2,3] facilities and healthcare workers have increased significantly. In war, there is the added potential complexity of receiving and treating contaminated casualties from the use of chemical, biological, or radionuclear weapons. An additional and distressing confounding factor has been the increasing use of rape and gender-based violence as tactics of war.

The disruption to social structures caused by conflicts and large-scale disasters, rapid urbanisation, population growth, and extreme weather events triggered by climate change have precipitated large-scale movements of people, both within and between countries. Such mass movements are often into already

DOI: 10.1201/9781003473718-4   25

insanitary and unsafe conditions that inevitably increase the risk of disease outbreaks and precipitate ever more complex humanitarian needs.

Set against these difficulties are improvements in technology, especially in healthcare, as a result of which we now have the ability to deliver high-quality healthcare in even the most austere environments. Point-of-care testing, portable battery-operated ultrasound, digital imagery, and many other advances all contribute to maintaining the standard of care provided to patients in these difficult circumstances. The simple mobile phone, almost ubiquitous now across the world, has made international consultations available to all, including video calls. Even when there is no mobile signal, although this is becoming rarer in an increasingly connected world, teams deploying to the remotest of areas can carry with them a handheld satellite telephone. As with everything, there are disadvantages. The use of mobile technology in a war zone brings with it a significant risk of location identity and consequent targeting. There are also international laws which must be obeyed when looking to transfer data across borders, particularly medical data.

There is no doubt that the advent of mobile phones, with their increasingly widespread coverage and data capacity, has improved the logistics of deployment and contact with, and within, the deploying team. A word of caution is needed, however, about the potential for 24-hour uninterrupted contact with those on deployment. Because contact is potentially continuous, gaps between phone calls can paradoxically increase anxiety amongst loved ones and trigger repeated, and potentially disruptive, calls from home to the field. It is better to agree on fixed times for daily contact, and when mobile phone contact is not available, for the organisation's HQ to agree with relatives on a daily update time.

If humanitarian assistance is to be as effective as it can be, teams and agencies must cooperate with each other. "*Competitive humanitarianism*", prompted by competition for a visible presence and fundraising publicity, is destructive and very wasteful of both human and material resources. There can be enormous pressure, either real or imagined, to be seen to be doing something in the eyes of those who have sponsored the team, but this must be resisted. Much useful work can be done away from the glare of publicity and in the support of the work of others.

The pressure to do something immediately can be considerable. Emotive television and press reports can galvanise public opinion into demands for immediate action, including by those who may be well-meaning but uninvited, and not always appropriately trained, experienced, or equipped to deploy. Without recognised terms of reference and a clear mandate to enter and work in another country, such teams may end up stranded at airports or otherwise adding to, rather than relieving, the logistical complexities of an already beleaguered nation. Those countries most in need of outside help may well have less robust systems for controlling who crosses their borders. It is incumbent upon the responders themselves, therefore, to ensure that their actions comply at all times with the four prima facie principles of good medical practice:[4]

- respect for autonomy (respect the patient's right to choose)
- beneficence (do good)
- non-maleficence (do no harm)
- justice (be accountable to your patient)

Medical teams must respect the autonomy of the patient, ensuring informed consent in their own language where necessary, and must be accountable to them through registration and authorisation to practice by the host government. They should be fully trained and experienced in working in humanitarian emergencies and practice only within their recognised competencies to ensure beneficence for their patients. Most major humanitarian organisations will only accept medical practitioners who are on the specialist or general practice register and will require at least five years post-qualification experience for other healthcare practitioners. Deploying personnel will also need comprehensive insurance, including medical indemnity insurance, just as they do at home. The victims of disasters and/or patients in low- or middle-income countries deserve justice and access to reparation no less than patients in high-income countries.

If an offer of help is accepted by the local authorities, time spent in securing a safe passage to the area involved and the identification of a task to be completed will result in a shorter journey to the scene and a more effective deployment. It is important that offered help should be in response to an identified need. *"Give what they ask for rather than what you have*" is a good maxim, and if what they need is not what can be offered, such a deployment may not be appropriate: available personnel may be better employed supporting the deployment of those who can meet the identified needs. The affected government will have carried out an assessment of needs, as will have large aid agencies and the UN through its United Nations Disaster Assessment and Coordination Team (UNDAC).[5] This will be discussed further in later chapters.

Before engaging in overseas deployment, it is essential to become familiar with the UN Cluster System.[6] This helps coordinate emergency relief, grouping areas of need into "clusters" of UN and non-UN agencies to which agencies can report and share information. The WHO is the lead agency for the Health Cluster alongside the local Ministry of Health. The cluster system is activated by the UN Emergency Relief Coordinator (ERC) (Under-Secretary-General for Humanitarian Affairs) at the request of the UN Resident/Humanitarian Coordinator. The UN agencies and their responsibilities are shown in Figure 4.1.

Whilst the timing of emergencies may be unpredictable, their consequences are usually not (Figure 4.2). It is imperative that teams are well briefed and prepared for the likely consequences of a particular type of event.

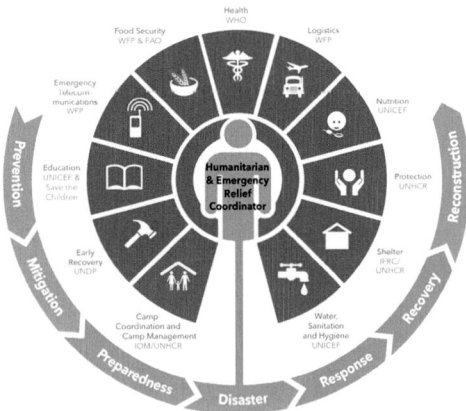

Figure 4.1 WHO agencies and responsibilities

Effect	Earthquakes	Strong Winds	Tsunamis and Flash Floods	Ordinary Floods	Landslides	Volcanic and Lava Activity
Loss of lives	High	Low	High	Low	High	High
Severe injuries requiring complex treatment	HIGH	MODERATE	LOW	LOW	LOW	LOW
Major risk of communicable diseases	Potential risk following all significant phenomena. Likelihood increases with crowding and degradation of sanitary conditions					
Damage to health facilities	Severe (structure and equipment)	Severe	Severe but localized	Severe (equipment only)	Severe but localized	Severe (structure and equipment)
Damage to water supply systems	Severe	Light	Severe	Light	Severe but localized	Severe
Food scarcity	Infrequent caused by economic or logistical factors)	(generally	Common	Common	Infrequent	Infrequent
Large migrations	Infrequent (common in severely affected urban areas)		Common (generally limited)			

Figure 4.2 Potential risks following natural phenomena

Equally important is an understanding of how the caseload is likely to change over time. If they are to survive, the majority of patients with life-threatening conditions will require treatment in the minutes and hours that immediately follow the onset of the disaster, which is often before even the most efficient international medical teams can arrive. Any immediate life-saving intervention will probably have been carried out by those present at the time or within no more than a few hours' travelling time of the disaster. Therefore, international teams, however quickly mobilised, will be unlikely to arrive in time to salvage those with severe head, chest, or abdominal injuries, but they can have an important role to play in the management of severe but not immediately life-threatening injuries, and certainly in supporting and assisting with complications of injury and reconstructive surgery.

However, coincidental emergencies will always continue to present to what is now a very stressed health system, where international medical assistance can be very important in supporting and maintaining the delivery of *essential emergency healthcare.* Maternal and child health in particular will always need support, and the WHO expects all medical teams that respond to have the capability of dealing with maternal and child health, including normal delivery and caesarean sections.

Just as good health is not entirely dependent on good healthcare alone and also requires political, social, and economic support, so effective emergency medical humanitarian assistance is equally dependent on a range of other inputs, most importantly the adequate supply of fresh clean drinking water and adequate sanitation, food, shelter, and security.

Those about to deploy or assist in the response to a humanitarian crisis must ensure that the team of which they are a part has the specific expertise and equipment that those affected are asking for. If this is not the case, it is usually better to give money than materiel. If drugs or medications are being donated, they must comply with all national and international regulations. Any deploying team must be fully self-sufficient. Appropriate supplies of water must be carried for the first two weeks until other sources have been identified by local or national agencies.

Clinicians must have secured or know how to obtain authorisation to practice in the host country. Team insurance must include full medical insurance, including repatriation coverage. Life insurance and medical indemnity insurance to cover the intended deployed activity must be in place. Finally, every member of the team must be familiar with the UN Cluster System and the EMT Coordination Cell. Humanitarian emergencies require well-equipped and experienced teams and are not the place for "backpack heroes".

NOTES AND REFERENCES

1. https://www.humanitariancoalition.ca/emergency-responses
2. https://www.who.int/activities/stopping-attacks-on-health-care
3. https://www.hcri.manchester.ac.uk/research/projects/current-projects/riah
4. Beauchamp, T. L., and Childress, J. F. Principles of Biomedical Ethics. 7th edition. Oxford University Press; 2013.
5. https://www.unocha.org/publications/report/world/undac-united-nations-disaster-assessment-and-coordination-system-2022
6. UNHCR. https://emergency.unhcr.org/coordination-and-communication/cluster-system/cluster-approach Cluster Approach

5

The Emergency Medical Teams (EMT) Initiative

Just as the response to the earthquake in Armenia in 1988 gave rise to a series of UN initiatives,[1,2] so concerns about the emergency medical response to the earthquake in Haiti in 2010 would give rise to the WHO Emergency Medical Teams (EMT) Initiative.

A failure by some in the past to recognise the importance of the principle of "*first do no harm*" when responding to sudden-onset disasters was one of the drivers behind the WHO and the Pan-American Health Organisation (PAHO) establishing and promoting a set of minimum core standards. In response to increasing international concerns about inadequately prepared and equipped medical teams responding to humanitarian emergencies, and especially the grave concerns about inadequate or inappropriate surgery by foreign medical teams that arose after the Haiti earthquake,[3] the WHO and the PAHO convened a 'meeting of experts' in Cuba in December 2010.

Out of this meeting came what was initially called the Foreign Medical Teams Working Group, the first task of which was to prepare and publish a classification and minimum standards[4] (the 'Blue Book') for what were now to be called *EMERGENCY MEDICAL TEAMS*, or EMTs. The classification would be similar to what was achieved by the INSARAG for search and rescue teams.

DOI: 10.1201/9781003473718-5

The work of the group expanded quickly to become the Emergency Medical Teams Initiative, with a permanent secretariat at the WHO in Geneva.[5] This led to the establishment of a set of minimum standards for deploying teams.

The EMT definition is intended to apply to everyone from very small groups of medical personnel to large professional teams from international and non-governmental organisations, and from governments. This definition can be applied to teams in or outside field hospitals, an important change from previous PAHO guidelines. It describes the services and people more than the facilities that they may or may not bring. EMTs are defined as:

> groups of health professionals and supporting staff aiming to provide direct clinical care to populations affected by disaster or outbreaks and emergencies as surge capacity to support the local health system. They include governmental (both civilian and military) and non-governmental teams and can be sub-classified as either national or international, dependent on the area of response.

According to the WHO, the purpose of the EMT Initiative is to improve the timeliness and quality of health services provided by national and international EMTs and enhance the capacity of national health systems in leading the activation and coordination of rapid response capacities in the immediate aftermath of a disaster, outbreak, and/or other emergency.

Integral to the EMT system is a classification system of emergency medical teams that mirrors a standard healthcare system of primary, secondary, and tertiary care facilities. This enables the affected country to more effectively choose the mix of healthcare support that it requires[6] (Figure 5.1 and Table 5.1).

EMTs must work in support of the national effort and not duplicate existing systems. By working through the UN/WHO channels they will ensure that they fit into the host national health system and can refer patients appropriately. Almost from the start of the deployment, the team must also be planning its exit strategy so patients can be appropriately and safely referred

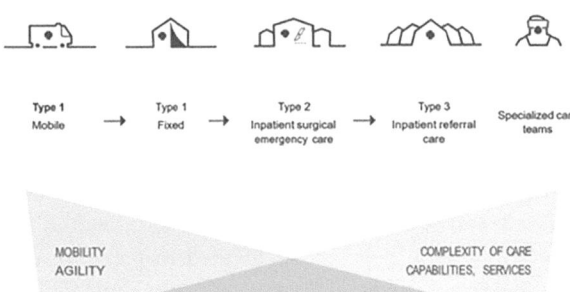

Figure 5.1 Levels of deployed humanitarian care (key in Table 5.1)

Table 5.1 Levels of Deployed Humanitarian Care (see also Table 5.2)

Type 1 Mobile	Provides daylight hours care for stabilisation of acute trauma and non-trauma presentations, referrals for further investigation or inpatient care and community-based primary care with the ability to work in multiple locations over the period of a deployment.
Type 1 Fixed	Provides daylight hours care for acute trauma and non-trauma presentations, referrals, and ongoing investigation or care and community-based primary care in an outpatient fixed facility.
Type 2 Inpatient surgical emergency care	Provides Type 1 services plus general and obstetric surgery, surgery for trauma and other major conditions as well as inpatient acute care.
Type 3 Inpatient referral care	Provides Type 2 services plus complex referral and intensive care capacity.
Specialised care teams	Additional specialised care teams that can be embedded in local healthcare facilities or Type 2 or Type 3 facilities unless specified otherwise, which can provide the following services: outbreak management, surgical, rehabilitation, mental health, reproductive and newborn care, interdisciplinary care, interhospital transfer, and technical support.

back into the local or national system that will continue to manage their care once the EMT has returned home.

It is essential that any help that is offered relieves rather than adds to the burden of the affected country. To that end, the EMT initiative expects teams to have been fully trained, to be fully equipped, self-sufficient in food water and medications for at least two weeks, and to have the experience and supply chains in place to replenish their stocks without draining the resources of the affected country. The WHO can verify teams as meeting the standards for their declared classification through a verification process that concludes with a team inspection. WHO verification allows affected countries to make more informed choices about outside medical assistance.

EMTs working in disasters are always required to keep medical records that comply with the national Ministry of Health (MoH) requirements for each patient and obtain informed consent from patients, in their own language, for all procedures. Each patient should be given a discharge summary in their own language, and teams can liaise with national and UN authorities if they need assistance with translation.

The process of EMT verification involves a request to the EMT secretariat and the allocation by the WHO of a mentor. The team then supplies the WHO with documentary evidence in support of their compliance with the core standards, which is followed by a site visit by the WHO and members of other already verified EMTs. Satisfactory completion of this process leads to global classification and verification (Figure 5.2).

On arrival, it is essential to work with the local authorities and within the framework they will be building, in order to ensure that work is focused on where it is most needed and does not unnecessarily duplicate the work of others. The UN is likely to have established a physical On-Site Operations Coordination

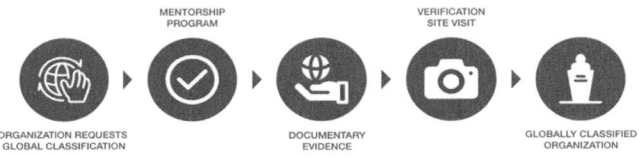

Figure 5.2 The verification and classification process

Centre (OSOCC), which is an important link between incoming humanitarian assistance and the host government authorities.[7] There will usually also be an online "virtual OSOCC" through which teams may make their offer of assistance and receive their invitation to deploy. Requests for and offers of assistance, including the types by classification of teams needed, are posted on the *virtual* OSOCC and matched by the WHOCC/MoH. On arrival in country, teams can be more efficiently dispatched to where they can be of most benefit.

The WHO will also have established an EMT Coordination Cell (EMTCC)[8] to which those EMTs they have invited into the country report on arrival, and then daily through its reporting system. The UN states that "Ideally, the EMTCC should be an entirely internal ministry of health entity (or a national authority equivalent) that is activated, managed and staffed by trained and experienced personnel from within the ministry of health". However, it recognises too that in many cases external support will be requested. Nevertheless, the primary responsibility for coordination will still remain with the national authority.

The scope of EMTCC activities can be divided into four broad areas:

- leadership and coordination
- communication with EMTs, the ministry of health, and other coordinating entities
- quality assurance
- operational support for the EMTCC

In order for countries requesting aid to rapidly gauge the type and capacity of the medical assistance that is being offered, the WHO EMT Initiative has established a classification system. Following a series of on-site visits, teams are verified as meeting the relevant minimum standard and capacity (Tables 5.1 and 5.2).

The development of the EMT classification and minimum standards process owes much to the experience of international search and rescue response operations and coordination, as developed by INSARAG,[9] which was established in 1991 with headquarters in the UN OCHA in Geneva. It established a peer

Table 5.2 Emergency Medical Teams (EMT) Capabilities and Capacities

Type	Capacity	Comments
Type 1 "mobile"	>50 outpatients a day	Providing remote area access teams for the smallest communities
Type 1 "Fixed"	>100 outpatients a day	Providing outpatient facilities +/− a tented structure
Type 2	20 inpatients >100 outpatients a day operating theatre	Capable of carrying out at least 7 major or 15 minor surgical operations daily
Type 3	40 inpatients >100 outpatients a day referral level care operating theatre high dependency care, including 4–6 intensive care beds	Capable of carrying out at least 15 major or 30 minor surgical operations daily
Specialist cell	Deploy into existing national facilities or into other EMTs to provide, for example, specialist surgical facilities, burns management, or rehabilitation.	

review classification system for *Urban Search and Rescue* (USAR) teams and common standards and coordination mechanisms that in many ways paved the way for EMTs.

In an emergency, it is critical to get the team with the right skills to the right place at the right time; therefore, the WHO's EMT classification list requires that all EMTs clearly outline their services and skills. Populations affected by disasters or public health emergencies need to be provided with quality healthcare by qualified professionals with established standards. The WHO EMT Initiative *requires* that all teams and their members are self-sufficient, registered specialists in their field, have suitable malpractice insurance, and are fully registered and authorised to practice by the national authority and lead international agency. They must declare the skills and services they will provide and report regularly to the relevant authorities during deployment. As stated earlier, they are required to maintain confidential patient records and establish agreed referral plans. It is imperative they work within the existing health system, ensure their supplies and medications meet all international standards, and they have established satisfactory hygiene, sanitation, and medical waste management. They must have a system in place care to for their team's health and safety, including repatriation if needed.

Once established in country there comes a consolidation phase. The team should assess:

- are we on the right track?
- are the right people doing the right jobs?
- is there a need for additional equipment and/or support?
- do we need to reconsider the distribution of workload?

How one leaves can be just as important as how one arrives. When intervening in a humanitarian emergency, it is imperative to plan one's exit from the time one arrives in order to provide continuity of care and to avoid the abandonment of those one has been treating.

NOTES AND REFERENCES

1. UNDAC—The United Nations Disaster Assessment and Coordination (UNDAC) system is managed by OCHA. OCHA mobilises UNDAC teams mostly in the event of a natural disaster, when a disaster-affected country requests international assistance and requires additional international coordination resources. OCHA also mobilises UNDAC teams in complex emergencies—when there is a sudden-onset emergency or a change in the intensity of a complex emergency that may need additional coordination resources. (unocha.org)

2. www.unsarag.org.uk
3. Redmond, A. D., et al. A Qualitative and Quantitative Study of the Surgical and Rehabilitation Response to the Earthquake in Haiti, January 2010. *Prehospital and Disaster Medicine*. 2011; 26: 449–456.
4. WHO Classification and Minimum Standards for Emergency Medical Teams. https://www.who.int/publications/i/item/9789240029330
5. https://www.who.int/emergencies/partners/emergency-medical-teams
6. https://www.who.int/emergencies/partners/emergency-medical-teams/emt-global-classified-teams
7. https://www.insarag.org//guidance-notes/manuals/v-osocc/
8. https://www.insarag.org//wp-content/uploads/2022/09/UC-Handbook-2022.pdf
9. https://www.insarag.org/

6

Armed Conflict and Complex Emergencies

Perhaps the biggest disaster of all is war. Armed conflicts precipitate major humanitarian emergencies, in the injuries they create and especially in the disruption they bring to society and to the delivery of healthcare. Women and children are particularly vulnerable, and a caesarean section, for example, is one of the commonest surgical operations to be carried out in a humanitarian crisis, even in a conflict zone.[1]

A complex emergency is defined as:

- a humanitarian crisis which occurs in a country, region, or society where there is a total or considerable breakdown of authority resulting from civil conflict and/or foreign aggression;
- a humanitarian crisis which requires an international response which goes beyond the mandate or capacity of any single agency;
- a humanitarian crisis where the IASC assesses that it requires intensive and extensive political and management coordination.[2]

There are several similarities between delivering humanitarian assistance in conflicts and sudden-onset disasters, and some very

DOI: 10.1201/9781003473718-6

significant differences. Medical support must obviously treat the wounds of war, but equally must compensate for the severe disruption to the pre-existing health system. This will require provision for treating coincidental emergencies, particularly obstetric emergencies, and the ongoing management of chronic conditions. There is, however, a significant difference. Unlike a sudden-onset disaster, where a single event precipitates an influx of casualties, medical teams working in conflicts must be prepared for repeated surges of patients as hostilities wax and wane (Figure 6.1).

The level of care that can be offered to patients is dependent very much on the maintenance of supply lines and evacuation routes. These are inevitably disrupted at times, sometimes continuously, during conflicts. If a patient cannot be safely evacuated up a referral chain to definitive care, then teams must consider carefully how far they should continue with resuscitation and interventions in an individual patient, knowing that the definitive care they need is not available in their forward station and evacuation is blocked. As is the case in emergency medical humanitarian assistance, the level of care offered to an individual and its impact on resources must be balanced against the broader standard of care that might be maintained if those same resources were distributed across a group or population.

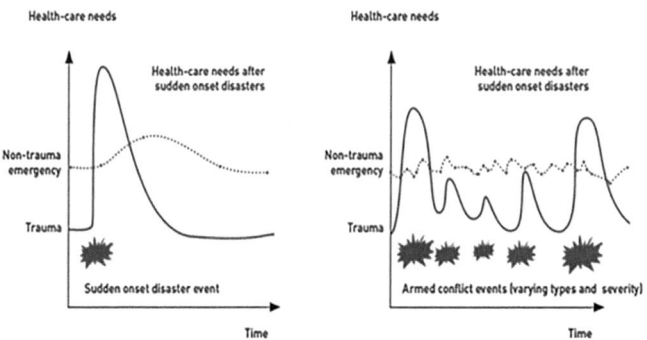

Figure 6.1 Healthcare needs differences after a sudden-onset event and during conflict

Delivering medical aid in a conflict involves another, special layer of complexity: the danger and significant threat to the lives of those involved in providing the care. It is incumbent on those who deploy humanitarian workers into conflict zones to take every step to mitigate the risks. It is also incumbent upon leaders in the field to constantly reassess these dangers and, if necessary, withdraw to an (often relatively) safer area. Individuals also have a responsibility not to put themselves or their colleagues, or indeed the mission as a whole, at unnecessary or avoidable risk. There can be a thin line between bravery and foolhardiness, and everyone involved must make sure that the benefits to patients are worth the risks being taken. Being there is not necessarily enough, although there is always potential value in bearing witness. Being there and making a difference is surely what counts the most. The risks for medical teams in responding to armed conflict can be very significant and cannot be eliminated, but they can be reduced by adequate preparation, increased awareness, and training.

Teams lacking the necessary preparedness, training, and supplies should consider not deploying at all, lest they harm themselves, the patients they seek to treat, and the confidence the warring factions and populations have in the care that is being provided. When a healthcare worker is killed or injured, it can mean not only the loss of an individual but the loss of the overall mission. Teams need to understand the context in which they are operating and the interaction between the intervention and its context, and act upon that understanding to avoid negative impacts and maximise the positive impacts of their actions on the conflict.

Working in conflicts can also raise ethical issues, particularly when trying to adhere to the humanitarian principles. Aid agencies may consider one party to the conflict to be in much greater need than another, or even the innocent victims of an unprovoked campaign of violence, but they must maintain their neutrality, impartiality, and independence. There is international humanitarian law to guide all parties, but when this is ignored, the already considerable difficulties faced by humanitarian agencies can only be compounded. Nevertheless, 'humanitarian' agencies must continue to position themselves within the 'humanitarian space' defined by the UN as "the operational environment that allows humanitarian actors to provide assistance and services according to humanitarian principles and in line with international humanitarian law and not align themselves with one party or another, perceived or otherwise", as perceptions can become distorted, either accidentally or deliberately. Agencies must be vigilant and continually reflect upon their work.

It is imperative that those who deploy understand the detailed background to the conflict and the position within it of those they are working alongside. Managing healthcare in such an environment requires a great deal of experience if interventions are not to be misconstrued or misrepresented and an already difficult situation made worse. There are guiding principles: just as in medical practice everywhere, adherence to the four principles of ethical medical care (respect for autonomy, beneficence, non-maleficence, and justice) must still be maintained along with technical standards and quality assurance. Importantly, there are international humanitarian law and humanitarian principles. When these are breached, particularly regarding impartiality, neutrality, and independence, then the very concept of a humanitarian space can be brought into question.

The key features of international humanitarian law demand that combatants must:

- not target people who are no longer engaged in the fighting;
- allow impartial humanitarian assistance to be given to the civilian population and all wounded and sick in general, including those who have previously taken a direct participation in hostilities ('*hors de combat*');
- not target those who are providing medical or humanitarian assistance;
- ensure that all wounded and sick receive medical care and the civilian population receive humanitarian assistance.

Emergency medical teams responding to conflict can look for guidance in the WHO 'Red Book'[3] (Figure 6.2), developed to be read alongside the 'Blue Book'.[3,4] In it will be found guidance on

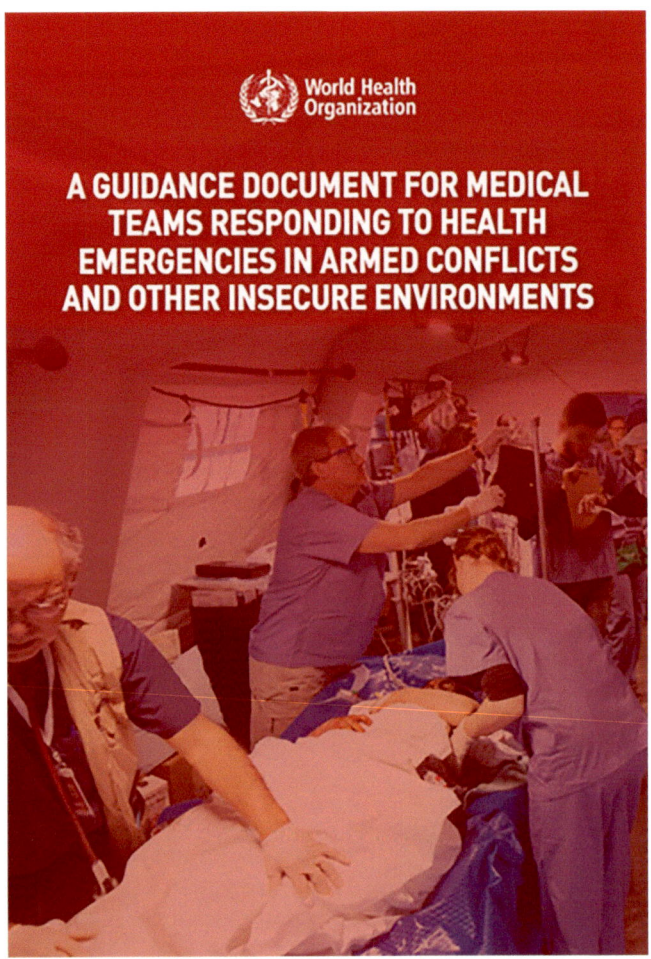

Figure 6.2 The Red Book

international humanitarian law and the application of the core humanitarian principles in the field. There is guidance on safety and security to complement and reinforce the security plans any deploying organisation must have in place and that all team members must understand before deployment. The classification criteria and verification processes described within the Blue Book are retained and expanded to accommodate the special circumstances encountered during conflict.

It is a tragedy that sexual and gender-based violence (SGBV) are features of modern warfare. There are detailed guides to managing these difficult presentations[5] with which all those working in conflicts must be familiar. While women are by far the most affected, men can also be victims. Patients require privacy and sensitivity with history taking focused only on what is required. A physical examination, including genito-anal examinations, will be required to determine what medical care is needed, but consent may be denied due to persisting mental trauma. Nevertheless, women or men who do not consent to a physical examination, or who are not able to complete the examination, must still be offered treatment, with an assurance of the strictest confidentiality. This treatment may include:

- treatment of physical injuries
- post-exposure prophylaxis (PEP) for HIV infection
- emergency contraception
- antibiotics for sexually transmitted infections (STIs)
- tetanus prophylaxis
- hepatitis B prophylaxis
- management of unintended/unwanted pregnancy

NOTES AND REFERENCES

1. https://www.msf.org/surgery-trauma-care
2. https://interagencystandingcommittee.org
3. A guidance document for medical teams responding to health emergencies in armed conflicts and other insecure environments. https://www.who.int/publications/i/item/9789240029354
4. See chapter 5.
5. https://www.unfpa.org/publications/briefing-paper-addressing-gender-based-violence-against-women-and-people-diverse

7

Deploying

Modern experience has shown that if emergency medical humanitarian assistance is to be of maximum benefit, and particularly if it is not to cause unintended harm, then those who respond must be well prepared, equipped, and practised.

However well intended, individuals or teams heading off to a disaster with small amounts of equipment and no previous experience can have minimal beneficial effect and are likely to place an unacceptable burden on already-stretched host facilities.

There is limited, if any, benefit in an individual deploying to a large-scale humanitarian emergency unless they have the specialist skills which have been specifically requested by a reputable organisation or health system and into which they will be assimilated. So those who wish to respond to the next humanitarian emergency should start their preparation at the earliest opportunity. This begins with joining a well-established and experienced humanitarian organisation. Most organisations require those who deploy to be fully qualified and registered to work independently.

Deploying into humanitarian emergencies requires a minimum degree of good health and fitness. A pre-deployment health screening including a self-declaration of existing and pre-existing medical conditions is usually required, often followed by a medical interview. Screening will often also include psychological assessment. The presence of common medical conditions is not usually of itself a barrier to deployment, as long as the condition is stable. This can be confirmed by the examining physician. What will have to be considered in any decision as to whether a team member is fit to deploy is whether the medication required

DOI: 10.1201/9781003473718-7

to treat that condition will be available in sufficient quantities for their deployment. Insulin is a case in point where a continuous, reliable, cold chain has to be guaranteed.

Pre-deployment training involves, amongst other things, written or online familiarisation with the organisation's policies and the UN cluster system. It will also involve a practical mock deployment exercise during which the team members become familiar with each other and the equipment they will be using. This usually involves putting up tented facilities and learning to work together. *'Whatever can be done by anyone is done by everyone'* should be embedded in the team, as well as *'what can only be done by a particular person is always done by that particular person.'* In this way, team members will learn to work as a team while acknowledging the special contributions of individuals.

The exercise will include a walk-through of the facility with a mock patient, explaining to the team the admission process, record keeping, and the progress through to, and location of, specialist departments.

One important exercise is to run through the management of a *mass casualty incident* (see Chapter 11: Triage). Not all members of the organisation will wish to deploy into areas of conflict. This should be respected. Those who have expressed a willingness to deploy into conflict must receive additional specialist training. This is most commonly provided through *hostile environment awareness training* (HEAT).

As well as becoming familiar with the team equipment, those who are to deploy must be familiar with the contents of their personal kitbag, which they will keep with them from the moment of deployment. Preparation for deploying into conflict areas may include specialist training in responding to chemical, biological, or radionuclear threats (CBRN).

BEFORE DEPLOYMENT

When dealing with any emergency, the better prepared one is, the better one will respond, and the better one will then recover from the event. Team members should be fully briefed regarding the work they are to carry out, only work within their qualifications and recognised competencies, and have been familiarised with the process of deployment. They should have been through a pre-deployment training course during which they become familiar with all the kit they will be taking or using, together with the range and limitations of the clinical procedures they will be expected to be able to perform. On deployment, each person will be given a kit bag with their personal first aid equipment (including trauma kit), sterile hand wipes, dressings, and antibiotics. Included will be a mobile phone, spare batteries, a torch or head torch, and a ration pack. It is important to include in one's personal bag a lightweight one-man tent, emergency blanket, sleeping bag, and bed roll. The journey to and from the humanitarian emergency can be very unpredictable, and it is essential to be prepared for unexpected, prolonged delays and stopovers. Depending on the deployment, a personal FFP2 face mask and intravenous giving set will be useful.

Teams must be familiar with how the field hospital or tented facility is unpacked and constructed. There will be team members whose primary role is to supervise and manage the process, but everybody will be required to assist.

As in all aspects of medicine, appropriate training should be completed before independent practice. The consensus view is that those preparing to deploy should have first completed their specialist training and then completed additional 'adaption' training for the humanitarian environment.[1] It is also important to have trained with colleagues and become familiar with the working environment and equipment, particularly if working in the unfamiliar environment of a tented field hospital. Pre-deployment "simulated deployments" help test and build teamworking and interpersonal skills (Figure 7.1). An essential component of this pre-deployment training is security training. Immediately before deployment, there may be an additional short training session on any special features or requirements, such as detailed PPE donning and doffing, training for deployment to an outbreak, or context-specific additional security briefings.

Pre-deployment training must include working in a tented facility and staying overnight in tented accommodation. Mass casualty simulation is very helpful, as is slow-time patient management simulation to enable team members to know what equipment

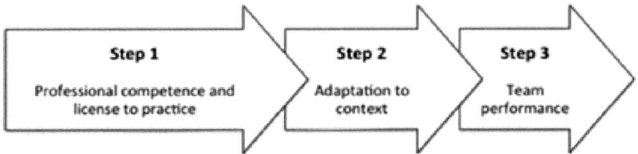

Figure 7.1 The three-step learning process for emergency medical teams

is available and where it is located. Surgeons in particular must understand that they will be working with standardised equipment and not necessarily have access to their preferred instruments.

DURING DEPLOYMENT

Teams function best when they are

- well protected
- well briefed
- well fed
- well watered
- well rested

Appropriate attention must therefore be given to safety and effective risk assessment, ensuring effective communication, both inside the team and to and from it. Adequate food and clean drinking water supplies must be available, and sensible rostering is essential to ensure adequate periods of rest.

POST-DEPLOYMENT

Deploying to any humanitarian emergency is a very intense experience, and returning to everyday life can be an enormous anticlimax. It is important that team members reunite with their loved ones as soon as possible, but they should be aware of the challenges of re-acclimatisation to the "normal". The team should be reunited as soon as possible in order that their experiences can be shared and better understood. Debriefing is best done in the form of a factual debrief where an individual's experiences are recounted and they hear the experiences of others. This is very similar to a team debrief after a major resuscitation. Individuals may be worried that they have misunderstood certain actions, and issues of this kind are often resolved following broader discussion and explanation. Similarly, they may consider their individual contribution to have been less than other team members, but when they understand what was achieved by the team as a whole, they are able to value the part they played. Immediate psychological debriefing has not been shown to be of benefit and can at times be harmful. It is better that individuals meet socially, and share their experiences, but for each member to look out for signs of stress in their colleagues. The organisation's occupational health team will usually do a follow-up telephone call with team members to explore any psychological difficulties and, when necessary, refer team members to professional psychological support.

LEADERSHIP

Making decisions in emergencies in the resuscitation room with an individual patient or in the middle of a humanitarian emergency requires individuals to act upon knowledge that is unfolding but not yet complete. This requires those in leadership roles to use their best judgement, draw on their knowledge and experience and all the information to hand, and then modify their decisions and directions to the team accordingly. This approach has been well summarised by General Colin Powell in his 40/70 rule. This states that you need between 40% and 70% of the total information required to make a good decision. With less than 40%, it is likely that a poor choice will be made, and with more than 70%, the decision may take too long and be overtaken by events, with the situation resolving itself adversely before a decision is made and implemented.

The point is that all leaders should aspire to make more correct decisions than incorrect ones. But they cannot be so fearful of making mistakes that they make no decisions at all. There has to be a balance between perfection and speed. It is important that team members do not lose faith in their leader when plans have to be changed according to the unfolding of events. The alternative is rigid adherence to a plan that is rapidly becoming out of date.

Dr Mike Ryan, Executive Director of the *WHO Health Emergencies Programme*, made a similar point during the COVID pandemic. He said publicly that "perfection [can be] the enemy of the good" in emergency management. "Speed trumps perfection", and "we must be fast". This was not a licence for recklessness or inappropriate or uninvited deployment, but rather of the need to have an understanding based on knowledge and experience that once the problem has been identified, "the greatest error is to be paralysed by the fear of failure". This is very similar to decisions made during a trauma resuscitation. It is clear that the patient has been injured, and a certain amount of information must be available before relevant interventions can be ordered, but waiting for every potential investigation to be complete may result in the patient dying from their as-yet-undiagnosed injuries. One has to make certain assumptions based on experience and training, for example about a potential tension pneumothorax or cardiac tamponade, and proceed accordingly. Importantly though, one must be prepared to change the direction of management as investigations reveal more about the nature and extent of the injuries suffered. It is the same during a large-scale emergency. Once the team has been asked to mobilise, speed is of the essence. It might be that on arrival in country it has become evident to local authorities that the scale of the disaster is such that it can managed by national facilities or enough international teams have already arrived. This is not a failure.

Leading others into danger is an awesome responsibility and requires absolute integrity. A leader must always be absolutely frank about the risks the team may face, and do everything to mitigate them. When briefing team members, the leader must address all the "what ifs?" Team members will want to know in particular what the plan is "if something happens".

Team leaders must also protect volunteers from themselves. Team members may underestimate the risks they face even with adequate preparation and planning. It is essential that leaders identify those vulnerable in this way and prevent them from overstepping the limits of their capabilities.

It must be made clear that volunteers are able to change their mind before deployment and up to and including the point of departure. It is imperative that this is impressed upon all team members, as changing their mind once deployed brings enormous difficulties for the team, although such choices have to be respected. When changing their mind, particularly prior to deployment, team members should understand that no explanation is required.

A leader must be:

- credible
- visible
- approachable
- collaborative
- inclusive

A perception by team members that the leader is holding things back or keeping secrets undermines trust. As a leader, it is important to be open about what one knows and honest about what one doesn't. If there is a reason for not sharing certain information, it should be given. The team will understand that there will be reasons for not sharing information, particularly in conflict, but should be reassured that they will informed as soon as possible and given the reasons why they could not be told at the time. Such circumstances, however, should be the exception and not the rule. The team must meet daily, ideally at a fixed time, even if nothing changes. Individual members of the team should only be asked to do what their leader would do themselves.

NOTES AND REFERENCES

1. Training for Deployment. Camacho, N. A., Hughes, A., Burkle, F. M., Ingrassia, P. L., Ragazzoni, L., Redmond, A., Norton, I., and von Schreeb, J. Education and Training of Emergency Medical Teams: Recommendations for a Global Operational Learning Framework. *PLOS Currents Disasters*. 2016, October 21; (1st Edition). PMID: 27917306. http://doi.org/10.1371/currents.dis.292033689

8

Needs Assessments

If aid is to do the most good for the most people, it must be targeted appropriately. To do this, a rapid needs assessment should be carried out as soon as possible, and in direct consultation with the host authorities. This may be done by the deploying team, or it may already have been done by international agencies working in tandem with the local authorities.

The United Nations OCHA developed two important initiatives following the earthquake in Armenia in 1988, when the huge outpouring of international assistance highlighted the need for better coordination of international offers of assistance and improvements in its quality assurance and standardisation. The United Nations Disaster Assessment and Coordination (UNDAC) team[1] was established by drawing on a range of international experts from across a variety of specialties and disciplines who could be mobilised at very short notice to deploy to the affected country and, by working with the relevant authorities, carry out a rapid *needs assessment* and disseminate its findings. This would facilitate a more targeted aid response, and with the establishment of an OSOCC,[2] the team would also help to coordinate the incoming humanitarian aid.

Reference has already been made to the INSARAG,[3] which was established at the same time to quality-assure the capabilities of search and rescue teams responding to large-scale disasters. Recognising that verifying the quality and relevance of offers of assistance in the immediate aftermath of a large-scale disaster would be extremely difficult and was likely to divert precious time and resources from the disaster itself, the international search and rescue community, working with the UN, established an advisory group to agree in advance of a disaster upon a set of general criteria and capabilities from which a classification system could be formulated (for example, light, medium, and heavy, depending on the type of equipment carried). Search and rescue teams could initially classify themselves against these criteria when offering assistance in order to guide the host government in choosing which teams to invite and where to deploy them in-country. INSARAG also established a training programme and a system of verification whereby the classification and capability of teams could be independently verified. In this way, affected countries could be assured of the quality and capability of search and rescue teams offering their assistance.

UNDAC TEAMS

The UNDAC team is a two- to six-person team drawn from member countries that travels quickly to a disaster scene, consults with local authorities, and establishes the immediate needs. These are then disseminated to the international community. UNDAC is a part of UN OCHA. It now serves as the international response system for sudden-onset emergencies, such as an earthquake or a flood, and it is designed to help the United Nations and governments of disaster-affected countries during the first phase of an emergency.

The fully self-sufficient team is deployed within 24–48 hours and can travel anywhere in the world. Its membership is drawn from professional and experienced emergency managers and humanitarian experts who have been made available by their respective governments or organisations to deploy alongside OCHA staff. UNDAC team members have been specially trained and equipped for this task.

EARLY ASSESSMENTS

It is critical to establish the presence or absence of

- safe drinking water
- adequate food supplies

- appropriate shelter
- sanitation and waste disposal
- medical care (and its complexity)
- the availability of essential items including blankets, heaters, water containers, and cooking facilities

People die of thirst long before they starve to death. Therefore, the greatest immediate threat is always from lack of adequate safe drinking water (potable water). Because humans require so much water, its quality must be balanced against its quantity: an adequate quantity of reasonably safe water is preferable to a smaller quantity of pure water. The recommended minimum maintenance requirements (including hygiene needs) are 15–20 litres per person each day. A feeding centre should aim to provide 20–30 l/person/day and a health centre 40–60 l/person/day.

In general, it is important to avoid "temporary" holding measures, which often fail to be replaced and become inadequate longer-term measures. For example, there are "temporary" refugee camps still in place years after they were first established. However, the urgency of supplying water is so great that temporary systems to meet immediate needs must often be installed, to be improved or replaced as soon as possible.

After water, the greatest need is adequate sanitation. Once again, the pragmatic provision of a basic system will save more lives than the delayed provision of a perfect system. There should be at least one latrine seat for every 20 people and with each dwelling no more than a minute's walk from a toilet. There will need to be at least one communal refuse pit for every 500 people, measuring at least 2 m × 5 m × 2 m.

The minimum maintenance level of food energy intake is accepted internationally as 2100 kcal (8.8 MJ) per person per day. When this falls below 1500 kcal (6.3 MJ) a day, mortality rises rapidly, especially in populations which are already poorly nourished. Locally prepared food with local ingredients is best received and therefore of greatest use. Moreover, the purchase of local ingredients by local and international agencies supports the local economy and is sustainable. If food cannot be obtained locally, then the provision of dried imported food still allows local preparation.

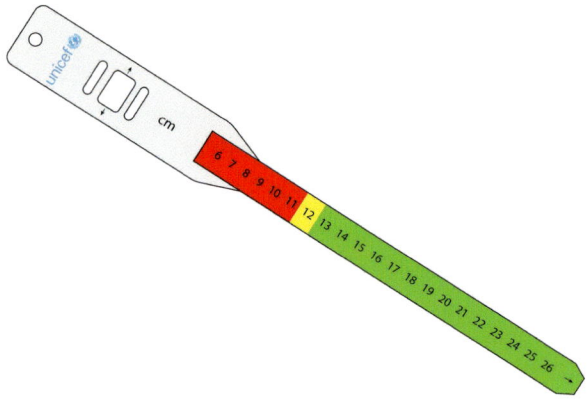

Figure 8.1 MUAC tape

The *middle upper arm circumference* (MUAC) in children aged under 5 years is a rough guide to nutritional status:

- normal > 14.0 cm
- moderate malnutrition 11.0–13.5 cm
- severe malnutrition < 11.0 cm

An emergency is declared when > 10% of children are classified as moderately malnourished.

MUAC is measured on the left arm, at the midpoint between the tip of the shoulder and the elbow. With the arm hanging straight down, a MUAC tape is applied around the arm and the value measured to the nearest 1 mm. A measurement in the green zone means the child is properly nourished, in the yellow zone that the child is at risk of malnutrition, and in the red zone that the child is malnourished (Figure 8.1).

When reporting the severity of a disaster, there are crude mortality rates that help convey this to international agencies and donors (Table 8.1). Trigger levels for urgent action include a rise in crude mortality of greater than 1/10,000/day and/or in children under 5 years old of more than 4/10,000/day.

The effects of the emergency on social infrastructure, particularly housing, must be assessed at an early stage and permanent shelter established as soon as possible. "*Temporary housing*" is rarely ever

Table 8.1 Assessing a Disaster by Mortality

Adults and children aged ≥ 5 years	Children aged <5 years
≤ 1* Under control	≤1 Normal in a developing country
>1 Serious condition	<2 Emergency under control
>2 Out of control	>2 Emergency in serious trouble
>4 Major catastrophe	>4 Emergency out of control

Source: *Mortality per 10,000 population per day

replaced and should be avoided whenever possible. The minimum floor area for a human to live in dignity is 3.5 m^2 per person.

It is always tempting to send clothing to disaster-stricken areas. It is rarely helpful: its transport is expensive, and its storage difficult and costly. It is almost always better to donate money to larger reputable agencies who will source goods locally, avoiding transport costs while simultaneously supporting the local economy.

Donations in kind can only be sent to those in need if they can be collected, dispatched, and delivered on time. Every team needs a strong logistics arm that can assess the logistical hazards on the ground, including the status and capacity of airports, seaports, and roads, and the availability of trucks and drivers.

When making an assessment of needs, it is essential to clarify and communicate which needs are immediate, which are medium-term, and which are longer-term. As already indicated, although the urge to give "things" to send people can be powerful, cash contributions will often best support the local economy by the employment of local people and the purchase of local goods and materials. A recommendation or decision to do nothing, either at all or at the present moment, can be a valid and helpful conclusion. If the local community is coping, the inappropriate or untimely dispatch of aid may only add to, rather than relieve, the burden of the affected country

REFUGEES AND REFUGEE CAMPS

The longer-term management of health conditions in humanitarian settings is well covered in MSF publications.[4] In refugee camps in particular, the most important medical issue will be infectious diseases. Children younger than 5 years are most vulnerable. WHO emergency health kits can be dispatched quickly and are available to match populations of varying sizes. Although primary care needs are paramount, limited support to secondary care is sometimes also appropriate.

WHO EMERGENCY HEALTH KITS

Basic and supplementary units are available and each unit is intended to assist a population of 10 000 for 3 months. The basic unit weighs 45 kg (0.2 m^3 in size), contains only oral drugs, and is meant for primary health workers. The supplementary unit weighs 410 kg (2 m^3 in size) and is for the sole use of health professionals. The supplementary unit does not duplicate the basic unit and cannot be used alone.

Although refugee camps are perceived as temporary solutions, many become permanent establishments. Everyone in a refugee camp is vulnerable, but women and children, the elderly, and the

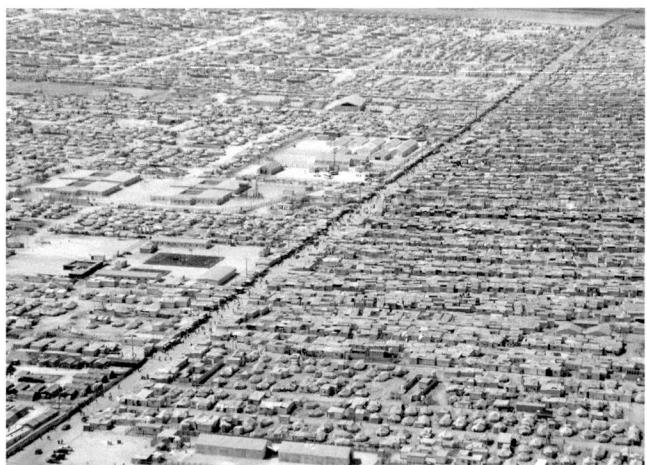

Figure 8.2 A section of the Zaatari refugee camp. Sited in Jordan and home to Syrian refugees, in 2018, the population housed about 78,000 refugees, of whom almost 20% were under five years old

disabled are particularly at risk (Figure 8.2). There is a special risk for women and young girls in regard to rape and sexual assault. This is exacerbated where toilet facilities are unlit and away from the main encampment. This must be considered when laying out a camp.

There will be an emergency phase following the arrival of refugees; this is the period during which mortality rates are higher than those experienced prior to displacement. This is defined by convention as when crude mortality rate (CMR) is above 1 death per 10,000 per day. The CMR in a stable population is around 0.5 deaths per 10,000 per day.

The post-emergency phase, or consolidation phase, is when mortality returns to the level of the surrounding population and the CMR is under 1 per 10,000 per day.

The ten top priorities in refugee camp health are

- initial assessment
- measles immunisation
- water and sanitation
- food and nutrition
- shelter and site planning
- healthcare in the emergency phase
- control of communicable diseases and epidemics
- public health surveillance
- human resources and training
- coordination[5]

NOTES AND REFERENCES

1. https://www.unocha.org/publications/report/world/undac-united-nations-disaster-assessment-and-coordination-system-2022
2. https://www.unocha.org/publications/report/world/site-operations-coordination-centre-osocc-guidelines-2018-enar
3. https://www.insarag.org
4. https://medicalguidelines.msf.org/
5. https://www.humanitarianlibrary.org//resource/refugee-health-approach-emergency-situations

9

Clinical Considerations

This book is not intended to describe in detail the management of specific clinical conditions. There are a number of established, practical courses[1,2,3] that comprehensively cover these issues, as well as detailed surgical texts and handbooks.[4] There are, however, some important general principles and adaptations that must be applied when managing trauma and other health conditions in humanitarian emergencies, and with limited resources. A particularly important concept to accept is that whatever care one perceives one's team to have deployed to provide, for example trauma care, the local population will always see the team simply as a medical facility to which they will present with whatever their health concern happens to be. It is essential, therefore, that all teams are prepared to respond to a wide range of medical presentations with immediate treatment protocols and onward referral pathways.

THE APPROACH TO TRAUMA AND SURGICAL CARE

It is important that the type of trauma care given has been appropriately adapted to the facilities in which the team is working and the constraints of the referral chain imposed by the wider impacts of the disaster. Resuscitation may be limited to life-saving initial care at the incident site or include advanced trauma life support, depending on the type of EMT facility. A type I outpatient

 DOI: 10.1201/9781003473718-9

team, for example, will provide triage and assessment of injuries with basic stabilisation of fractures, wound cleaning, and immediate discharge or onward referral of patients who require general anaesthesia to a type II or type III facility. Generally, in disasters, any procedure that can be carried out under local or regional anaesthesia should be, with general anaesthesia reserved for those cases where there is no alternative. Type II and type III facilities will deliver in-patient trauma care with wound debridement, closed fracture management with splintage and external fixation, and damage control surgery. Internal fixation is not recommended in these circumstances, as the risk of post-operative infection is too high. It is important that the medical team ensures that appropriate follow-up for patients is established, for example for the removal of external fixation.

There are established protocols for wound care in these environments, such as those developed by the ICRC. The key principles involve effective wound toilet, debridement, and delayed primary closure; the wounds inevitably involve an element of crush and contamination. In a type II or III facility, surgical capacity must extend to the construction of basic flaps and skin graft procedures to cover wound defects following debridement. Amputation is discussed below.

Reconstructive surgery is an important feature of the surgical response after earthquakes in particular, and can be incorporated within the EMT itself or by the deployment of a specialist reconstructive surgical team to augment another EMT or a local health facility. There are specialist burns management teams that deploy to disasters involving large numbers of burned patients. However, the management of individual burns must be within the competence of all EMTs.

Whether in a tent or in a more substantial facility, all EMTs carrying out surgery have to meet the minimum standards for instrument sterilisation as laid down in the WHO EMT Blue Book, with thorough cleansing of instruments followed by steam sterilisation or autoclaving between every case.

Pharmacy and medicines management are core elements of an EMT and ensure appropriate and safe prescribing. The WHO model list of essential medicines is a good guide to generic medicine supplies for EMTs, but additional specialist medications will be required, for example, when responding to disease outbreaks. If pharmaceuticals and/or equipment are to be donated when the team leave the country, this must be done with the knowledge and consent of the local MoH, and drugs and disposables must be at least 1 year from their expiry date or meet the requirements of the national MoH.

Advances in technology mean that even in a field hospital, adequate imaging can be facilitated. At the very least, a portable ultrasound machine should be part of the equipment, although many teams also take portable X-ray facilities. Similarly, point-of-care testing has greatly improved the laboratory support available to EMTs responding to a sudden-onset disaster (Table 9.1).

If available, the X-ray imaging tent should be located at the end of the field hospital site. There should be adequate signage to clearly identify its function and the tent should be clearly marked with brightly coloured warning tape or rope to form a surrounding boundary at 5 metres distance. Lead aprons must be provided to protect staff and patients from radiation exposure.

The required range of surgical skills required is broad. They are often not present in a single individual or contained within a single subspecialty training programme, so additional training to broaden surgical expertise is recommended. One such course is the Hostile Environment Surgical Training United Kingdom (HEST-UK) at the Royal College of Surgeons of Edinburgh. Some teams may be able to accommodate the breadth of surgical expertise required by incorporating a number of individual specialists into the team. However this is achieved, teams will be expected to treat surgical cases in both adults and children, as well as surgical emergencies unrelated to the disaster.

Obstetric emergencies in particular require that each team has the capability to carry out a caesarean section safely and, if required, is able to support the local health service by relieving some of the burden of routine surgery, particularly non-disaster-related surgical emergencies. Figure 9.1 shows approximate timelines for different elements of clinical care following a sudden-onset disaster.

Table 9.1 Essential Laboratory Tests

Type 1 EMT	Type 2 EMT	Maternity Tent
Blood glucose	**i-Stat CHEM8+**	Rapid Syphilis test
Rapid single test for pregnancy	• Sodium (Na)	(Maternal and Accidental Exposure ONLY)
Urinalysis	• Potassium (K)	Rapid HIV Antibody test (1st and 2nd)
Haemocue (Hb)	• Chloride (Cl)	(Maternal and Accidental Exposure ONLY)
Malaria Rapid Single Test	• $(total)CO_2$	Rapid Hep B and C test (Accidental Exposure ONLY)
	• Anion Gap	
	• Ionised Calcium	
	• Glucose (Glu)	
	• Urea Nitrogen/Urea	
	• Creatinine	
	• Haematocrit (Hct)	
	• Haemoglobin	
	• HCO_3	
	i-Stat: CG4+	
	• Lactate	
	• pH	
	• PCO_2	
	• PO_2	
	• $(total)CO_2$	

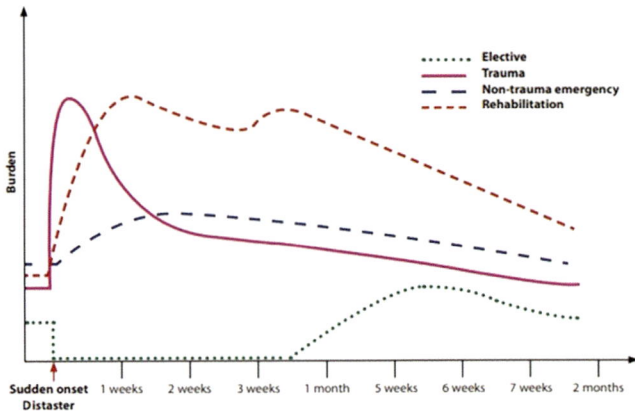

Figure 9.1 Approximate timelines for different elements of clinical care following a sudden-onset disaster

BASIC CLINIC PRINCIPLES

Wound Management

Wounds of all shapes, sizes, and severities are common in the humanitarian setting, and there are some basic rules which should be followed, or broken only with good reason. The following basic principles apply:

- all war wounds are contaminated wounds.
- all crush injuries are contaminated wounds.
- all wounds older than a few hours are contaminated wounds.
- healing is by delayed primary closure.

The surgeon must first assess the level of contamination and identify and remove all devitalised tissue. Aggressive cleaning and debridement follow a full assessment with continuous and adequate analgesia (type 1 and 2 facility) or, if required, anaesthesia (type 2 and 3 facilities only) being maintained throughout. Foreign bodies should be removed and the integrity of underlying structures confirmed by wound extension and further exploration, if required. Irrigation

Table 9.2 Principles of Wound Management
- initial adequate debridement
- wound dressing
- careful wound reassessment at 48 h
- repeat debridement and dressing if necessary
- closure at 48 hours or longer after the initial inspection and only if the wound is clean and free of foreign material, contamination, and devitalised tissue
- simple closure techniques are preferred including Steri-strips®, sutures, or staples, all of which should be used to bring the wound edges together without undue tension
- wounds that cannot be closed without tension should be left open to heal by secondary intention or closed by a skin graft or flap (if the environment is appropriate)
- complex wound closure may require onwards referral to a Type 3 facility

of wounds can be carried out with isotonic saline, distilled water, boiled and cooled water, dilute antiseptic solution, sterile water, or drinkable (tap or potable) water, all of which have similar efficacy. The use of dilute antiseptics, such as 1% povidone–iodine or a 5% solution of sodium benzyl penicillin, can decrease infection rates and may be used in addition to water or normal saline.

Delayed primary closure follows the sequence shown in Table 9.2. The dressing should be kept simple. An absorbent gauze dressing or saline-soaked gauze dressing and coverage with dry gauze is sufficient.

Anaesthesia

Wherever possible, procedures should be carried out under local anaesthesia; more complex procedures can be done under regional anaesthesia (and therefore teams should ensure that they have the appropriately skilled staff and equipment). Spinal anaesthesia offers an alternative, but again the skills and equipment must be available within the team. Unfortunately, spinal anaesthesia requires a level of patient supervision that may not always be available. The use of general anaesthesia should be limited given the personnel and equipment it requires, but there will inevitably be cases where it will have to be used. Whilst the technical difficulties of transporting anaesthetic gases in an aircraft are not insurmountable, most international teams restrict general anaesthesia to total intravenous anaesthesia.

Antibiotics

These are indicated for wounds at high risk of infection; this includes the majority of wounds seen in humanitarian emergencies, which are almost inevitably contaminated. Other high-risk wounds include penetrating wounds, abdominal trauma, compound fractures, lacerations larger than 5 cm, and wounds with devitalised tissue. Special consideration should also be given to high-risk anatomical sites such as the face, genitalia, hands, and feet.

With all wounds, attention must be directed towards tetanus prevention. The primary preventive measure is adequate initial wound care, including debridement and removal of dead and damaged tissue. In those known to be vaccinated, a tetanus toxoid booster can be given. In those unvaccinated and with high-risk wounds, anti-tetanus serum must be considered as well as tetanus toxoid vaccine, given using separate syringes and at different sites. Anti-tetanus serum should be considered in patients presenting with wounds already older than 12 hours and/or with heavy contamination.

Blood Transfusion

Blood for transfusion is usually not available, or is at least very restricted, in large-scale disasters. Local facilities may still be functioning, but the demands on their supplies will quickly deplete their stocks. International agencies such as the WHO will look to establish blood transfusion facilities in support of international medical teams, but this inevitably takes time to be fully functional. Incoming teams will not have the facilities to safely store and carry blood supplies from their home country, but must have the equipment and skills to group and crossmatch blood. In military practice especially, whole blood may be harvested from deployed personnel who as part of their pre-deployment screening will know their blood group and have been screened for hepatitis and other blood-borne diseases. This practice is known as a '*walking blood bank*'. It has the potential to be used in civilian deployments for the treatment of catastrophic haemorrhage, where the risks of transfusion reaction even in the presence of ABO compatibility are outweighed by the threat to the life of the patient. Deployed team members should know their ABO blood type and have been screened for the detection of *transfusion transmittable diseases* (TTDs), such as hepatitis B, hepatitis C, HIV, and syphilis. However, as only one unit of blood per volunteer can safely be harvested, in practice it is rarely used. Blood donations may also be harvested from volunteer team members whose blood group has already been established prior to mobilisation. There are rapid tests for ABO/Rh blood typing, and rapid testing is available for HIV (human immunodeficiency virus), HCV (hepatitis C virus), HBsAg (hepatitis B surface antigen), syphilis, and malaria.

Catastrophic events such as massive haemolysis due to ABO mix-ups or anaphylactic reactions usually become apparent after a very small amount of blood is transfused. The more rapidly these are detected, the more rapidly the blood can be discontinued and treatment instituted. If no problem occurs in the first 5–15 minutes, the risk of immediate life-threatening complications declines sharply, although it can still occur.

COMMON CLINICAL PROBLEMS

Head Injuries

The limitations placed on the surgical management of head injuries are determined by the level of surgical facilities, the skills and experience of the operator, the availability of adequate supplies of blood for transfusion, and the capacity for prolonged mechanical ventilation. Not all of these will be present in an emergency field hospital or in emergencies with limited resources. This is why the potential for head injury management in a humanitarian emergency is usually limited to non-operative, non-ventilatory care. Uncomplicated scalp wounds can be debrided, irrigated, and closed under local anaesthesia. If there is an underlying skull fracture, the wound can still be closed, but great caution must be exercised where there is a comminuted fracture in order to ensure that fragments are not dislodged and damage underlying tissues. Small, depressed fractures are best left alone, as attempts at elevation may again damage underlying tissues and precipitate catastrophic haemorrhage.

Exploring deeper than the skull vault is generally not advised, again to avoid the risk of provoking or precipitating uncontrollable haemorrhage. In the absence of CT imaging, usually the case in these circumstances, extra- or sub-dural haemorrhages cannot be diagnosed with any degree of certainty. Exploratory burr holes guided by clinical presentation may be a theoretical consideration, but in practice in these settings are likely to be unfruitful and are risky.

A key decision in resuscitative interventions is what happens when success is not immediate or the patient does not wake up. Teams that respond to humanitarian crises will inevitably have limited resources. This is particularly so in the case of ventilators, which will be prioritised for use in emergency surgery where other anaesthetic techniques cannot be used. Elective ventilation of severe head injuries is almost invariably not possible. It may be considered appropriate to do this in an existing facility whose resources have been preserved, but such decisions require a balance between likely outcome and the diversion of resources. For these reasons, endotracheal intubation of patients in humanitarian crises is uncommon, and resuscitation limited to temporary bag and mask ventilation.

Severe Haemorrhage

Penetrating injuries to the chest and abdomen with corresponding severe haemorrhage will require rapid intervention if lives are to be saved. Given the short time it takes to bleed to death from such injuries, it is those already at, or near, the scene who will provide life-saving interventions. For this reason, incoming international teams after an earthquake will rarely have to manage these cases as they simply arrive too late. It is crushed soft tissues and fractures that will form the majority of their surgical workload. However, teams responding to conflicts which usually involve repeated outbreaks of hostilities *will* need the skills and equipment to manage such injuries. The success or otherwise of surgical intervention will be limited by the availability of intravenous fluids and especially blood for transfusion.

Crush Injury

Whilst the primary aim of surgery is always to preserve tissue, attempts at muscle salvage can become futile in limbs that have been crushed for a prolonged period and are showing evidence of extensive devitalised muscle. Bleeding and extravasation of fluids from crushed tissues produces swelling which, in the confined space of tissue compartments, leads to increasing pressure that compresses blood vessels, leading to tissue ischaemia and ultimately necrosis—*compartment syndrome.* Pressure can be relieved by performing a fasciotomy: cutting through the fascia to relieve this pressure. However, this procedure carries its own risks of bleeding, wound infection, and sepsis. A careful risk/benefit analysis must be undertaken which emphasises the importance of experienced trauma surgeons deploying to these emergencies.

The presence of crush injuries, particularly when surgical treatment is delayed, increases the risk of *crush syndrome.* This occurs when the products of muscle breakdown are released into the circulation and cannot be adequately filtered by the kidneys with ensuing renal failure. Septicaemia can also accompany these phenomena. Effective treatment requires early and aggressive intravenous fluid therapy hydration. Forced alkaline diuresis may be of benefit but the evidence is currently not conclusive. This requires additional specialist knowledge and such patients should be referred onwards to specialist units and certainly a facility that can ultimately offer haemodialysis. Such facilities are obviously in limited supply in the circumstances of a disaster, emphasising the importance of prevention of crush syndrome by adequate debridement and early intravenous fluid therapy.

Amputation

Careful consideration must be given to the role of amputation. Amputation of a limb under any circumstances is a major decision for both patient and surgeon and will inevitably produce some degree of disability. The disability imposed by the loss of a limb for someone already living in impoverished circumstances is considerable. Even if supplied with a prosthesis by the initial team, the chances of the patient being able to replace it can be small. There can also be a social stigma associated with amputees in some cultures. Therefore, the aim of surgical intervention when limbs have been damaged, particularly in earthquakes and conflicts, is to preserve limbs—either in their entirety or with as much length as possible. EMTs should therefore try and preserve limbs and limb-length as much as possible, and so are required to have an appropriately trained surgeon in their team when responding to emergencies where amputation is likely to be required. Guillotine amputations are no longer an acceptable surgical procedure and should be avoided. Decision-making in these circumstances can be facilitated by reference to the *Mangled Extremity Scoring System (MESS)* (Table 9.3) and consensus guidelines.

Immediate amputation, even in the most dire of circumstances, should be relatively unusual. It may be that those trapped can only be freed by amputation of a limb, but this is a relatively rare event. More commonly the surgical intervention at the scene is only to complete what has more or less already been achieved by falling masonry or ballistic injury. Similarly, patients may present to a medical facility with an established partial amputation that requires completion. Of course, if transfer to an adequate treatment facility has been very much delayed then advanced tissue necrosis, irreparable vascular injury, or sepsis may make immediate amputation unavoidable. Amputation of a mangled or devitalised limb should only be performed by a suitably qualified surgeon and after they have carefully evaluated the limb. Teams should have included a rehabilitation specialist and ensured their early involvement.

Table 9.3 The Mangled Extremity Severity Score (MESS). A Score of 6 or Less is Consistent With a Salvageable Limb. If the Score is 7 or More, Amputation is the Usual Eventual Outcome.

Skeletal/Soft Tissue Injury	Score
Low energy (stab, simple fracture, pistol GSW)	1
Medium energy (open or multiple fractures, dislocation)	2
High energy (high-speed MVC or rifle GSW)	3
Very high energy (high-speed trauma with gross contamination)	4
Limb ischaemia	
Pulse reduced or absent but perfusion normal	1*
Pulseless, paraesthesia, increased CRT	2*
Cool, paralysed, insensate, numb	3*
Shock	
Systolic BP always >90mmHg	0
Transient hypotension	1
Persistent hypotension	2
Age	
<30	1
30–50	2
>50	3

Source: *Double the score in cases of ischaemia >6 hrs
GSW gunshot wound; MVC motor vehicle collision; CRT capillary refill time

Burns

Collapsed buildings can damage electricity and gas supplies, which in turn may lead to fires. Detonation of explosive ordnance may cause burns as well as causing the collapse of buildings. Improvised cooking facilities can be lethal. As a result, burn injuries are not uncommon in humanitarian emergencies, either alone or complicating other injuries. Their management follows that of all injured patients. In addition, there is the risk of inhalation burns with corresponding rapid airway compromise. Fluid loss can be considerable and must be managed. The swelling of burned tissues also raises the risk of compartment syndrome.

It is important to estimate the percentage area of burned tissue and its depth. There are established charts to help in this assessment, such as the rule of 9s for adults and the "rule of 5s" for children (Figures 9.2 and 9.3). A quick assessment can be carried out using the palm of the patient's hand as a representing roughly 1% of their surface area.

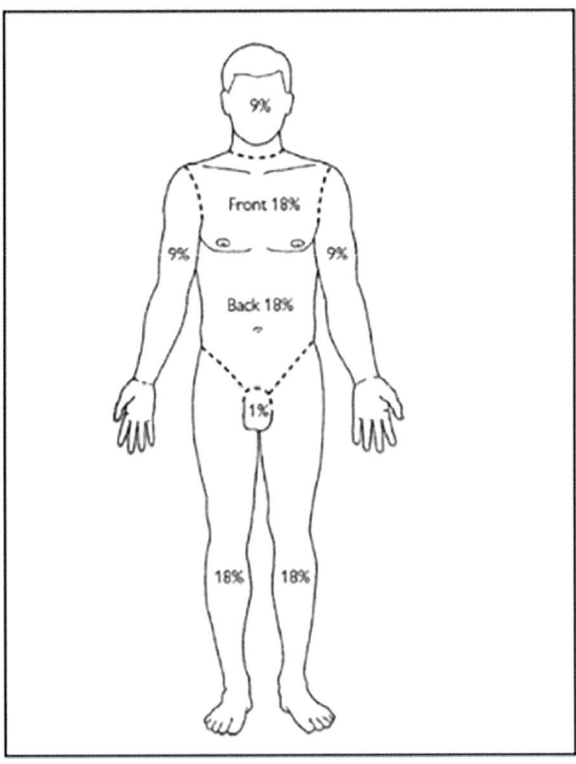

Figure 9.2 The rule of 9s

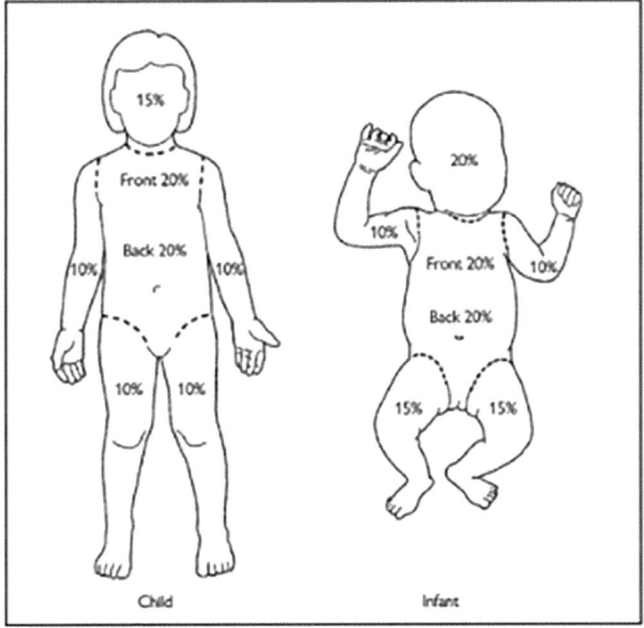

Figure 9.3 The rule of 5s

Burned tissues retain the heat of burning which continues to cause damage. If the patient arrives at the health facility without first aid having been given, all burned clothing must be removed and the burn should be drenched thoroughly and continually with cool clean water to prevent further tissue injury. With smaller burns, the site can be immersed in cold water for 30 minutes to reduce pain and oedema, as well as limit further tissue damage. Larger burns should be doused with cool water, and then clean dressings or coverings applied to the burned area to prevent systemic heat loss and hypothermia as well as to reduce pain. Tetanus prophylaxis must not be forgotten. For those burned patients who remain under the EMT's care, burns should be dressed with petroleum gauze and dry gauze thick enough to prevent seepage to the outer layers. The dressings should be changed regularly under adequate analgesia/anaesthesia.

FRACTURE MANAGEMENT

Fractures are dealt with as simply as possible and along conventional lines. The initial management is to reduce the fracture and realign the deformity and thus reduce pain and control bleeding. The limb can then be immobilised in a splint. Splintage will reduce the risk of neurological and vascular injury and possible further tissue damage as well as reducing pain. It is important to assess and document the distal neurologic and vascular status of the limb, both before and after realignment and splinting.

With open (compound) fractures, the absence of internal compression increases the risk of significant haemorrhage which must be controlled as rapidly as possible by placing a sterile pressure dressing over the injury site. All patients must receive adequate pain relief by whatever route is most appropriate.

In sudden-onset disasters and conflicts an obvious fracture may not of course be the only injury, and it is important to carry out a full assessment of the patient, following traditional ABCDE protocols. Resuscitation when required will precede more complex fracture management though adequate splintage can help control haemorrhage. It is important not to be distracted by the obvious injury and to carry out a full inspection of an undressed patient. In conflicts, care must be taken when undressing combatants as they may be carrying weapons and ordinance.

Most fracture reduction will be achieved by closed manipulation, although if the facilities and expertise are available, and in practice these will be restricted to a type 3 field hospital/EMT, then open reduction can be considered. Traction is then applied. Maintenance of alignment is achieved by splintage, including casting, and by the application of external fixators.

Although internal fixation is usually required for comminuted, displaced, intra-articular, or complex fractures with joint incongruity, this can be very difficult to perform safely in a field hospital. If teams are deployed into existing hospital facilities with good laminar flow, then the risk of infection can be reduced sufficiently to consider this degree of intervention. However, it is not usual practice in field hospitals where laminar flow is usually not available. Conservative immobilisation can be used for most fractures, either as treatment in itself or to stabilise factures before reduction or fixation can be performed.

Prior to the establishment of minimum standards by the WHO EMT Initiative, inadequate sterilisation of surgical instruments by incoming medical teams was one of the major concerns voiced by the international medical community. Proper decontamination and sterilising of re-usable surgical equipment is essential. The first and most important step involves the cleaning of instruments by the physical removal of contaminants followed by thorough drying. This is followed by disinfection, using heat or chemicals, to reduce the number of viable micro-organisms to a level which is not harmful to health. This will not remove all viruses and/or bacterial spores. The final stage is sterilisation, to render the instruments free from viable micro-organisms, including bacteria, spores, and viruses.

MENTAL HEALTH

Patients in acute psychological distress can present to emergency medical facilities. All team members should be aware of the concept of *Psychological First Aid* (PFA).[5,6] PFA aims to provide non-intrusive practical care and support designed to assess needs and concerns. It is normal for people to be distressed in these circumstances, and help with basic needs such as food and water can be a great comfort. Simply allowing people to talk without pressure as well as providing words of comfort can be both calming and reassuring. It is of course important not to overpromise, but where possible to connect people to reliable sources of information and social support and when necessary to try to protect them from further harm.

PFA is not something that only professionals can do, and it is not professional counselling. Importantly, it is not "psychological debriefing", and it does not necessarily involve a detailed discussion of the event that caused the distress or asking someone to analyse what happened to them. Although PFA does involve being available to listen to people's stories, it is not about pressuring people to open up about their feelings and reactions to an event. If such interventions are thought necessary, then so is

Table 9.4 Elements of Psychological First Aid
- making initial contact with the patient
- ensuring people are safe and comfortable
- calming and orienting people
- identifying people's immediate needs
- offering practical assistance
- connecting people with the resources they need
- providing coping strategies
- linking people to the services they need

referral to psychiatric/psychological expertise. Similar techniques can be used to support colleagues (Table 9.4).

Patients in acute psychosis can present to the field hospital and should be guided to a calmer, more private area of the facility where, with the help of interpreters, they can be reassured while a history is taken directly from them or from those who have accompanied them. If the degree of agitation is such that sedation is required, this should be, whenever possible, with their informed consent. If their behaviour is such that they are a serious threat to themselves or others, the senior clinician on duty must discuss with colleagues and those who accompanied the patient whether temporary sedation without their consent is justified. For patients who are relatively mildly agitated, oral diazepam can help, but more agitated patients might require oral haloperidol and severely agitated patients intramuscular haloperidol.

THE MANAGEMENT OF NON-COMMUNICABLE DISEASES

The disruption to the provision of healthcare services caused by large-scale sudden-onset disasters and conflicts will have a profound effect on those with chronic conditions and the presentation of recent-onset medical diseases.

It is important to appreciate that whatever purpose is envisaged for the field hospital or facility, including a focus on trauma, patients with a variety of needs will present to any medical facility they perceive to be offering assistance. Those responding to humanitarian emergencies must be able to manage a range of conditions and not just trauma.

The safe management of diabetes, for example, requires a continuous supply of oral medication or insulin. The supply of insulin in particular raises significant logistical problems in humanitarian emergencies, as its safe storage and transport requires continuous refrigeration. Asthma and hypertension are common worldwide, and patients may lose their medication in the destruction associated with the disaster or be separated from it as they flee from conflict.

Emergency medical teams responding to any humanitarian emergency must be able to provide at least a limited supply of common medications to those who present to their facility, as well as working with local health authorities, UN agencies, and the WHO to ensure further supplies. Given the likely time limits of deployment, emergency medical teams will be unable to provide ongoing or continuing care to those with long-term chronic health conditions. It is also important that teams do not replace or override the host country's own health service provisions. However, teams must be able to deal with any immediate patient needs, particularly in the provision of rescue medication, and manage any urgent exacerbations or complications of chronic diseases and the consequences of missed doses. Patients can then be referred on to the relevant national/in-country long-term health provider.

Diabetes

Pre-coma hypoglycaemia can often be managed with the administration of sugary drinks. Hypoglycaemia is managed with the administration of 50 ml of 10% glucose intravenously or, if intravenous access is difficult, intramuscular glucagon via injection kit.[7] Diabetic hyperglycaemic patients require resuscitation with intravenous fluids and repeated small doses of insulin while the blood glucose and electrolytes are regularly monitored until the vital signs are stable. If the patient has run out of their medication, this can be replaced and the patient allowed home; otherwise, arrangements should be made for onward referral and follow-up.

Asthma and COPD

If the patient is not in severe respiratory distress, their peak flow should be measured and they should be given a salbutamol inhaler with instructions for its use. The peak flow measurement can then be repeated. All patients with asthma should be referred on to a facility that can replace their medication when required and arrange their follow-on care. If the patient has simply run out of medication but is not in any distress, they should be referred on to a facility that can replace their medication and arrange follow-on care.

Amongst patients presenting with exacerbations of *chronic obstructive pulmonary disease* (COPD) and other chronic lung diseases, intercurrent infection is the likeliest cause of an exacerbation; it can be treated with oral antibiotics and the patient given a 5-day supply to take home. Arrangements for long-term follow-up in a more appropriate facility should be arranged.

Hypertension and Cardiovascular Disease

Hypertension is common and patients may have run out of their medication or lost access to it during emergency. It is important to reconnect patients with an ongoing facility that can provide continuing care. The blood pressure should be measured and if clinically indicated a 5-day supply of an antihypertensive agent may be given to the patient but linked to establishing referral to an ongoing treatment facility. Patients with other cardiovascular diseases, including angina, should be assessed clinically and when stable, referred on to a facility that can provide ongoing care.

Musculoskeletal Problems

Increasing pain and reduced mobility are the commonest non-urgent presentations. The patient's medication should be reviewed, and where necessary they should be provided with a 5-day supply of paracetamol and/or ibuprofen and referred on to a facility that can provide ongoing care. In addition, patients can be assessed by the rehabilitation specialist within the team who can, if required, prescribe orthoses and other aids.

HIV/AIDS

The most likely cause of a deterioration in the patient's condition will be lack of access to their regular antiretroviral medication with or without intervening infection. The patient should be assessed and a limited supply of antiretroviral therapy provided with appropriate antibiotic medication if required. They will require onwards referral to a facility that can provide ongoing care.

Tuberculosis (TB)

Patients with TB are likely to present because they have run out of medication, and the presentation may also be associated with underlying HIV/AIDS. Potentially infectious patients must be isolated while a referral to the local TB clinic is arranged.

Cancer

Patients already diagnosed with cancer may present for additional medication, a second opinion, or a request for surgery. Emergency medical teams are not set up to carry out surgery for cancer, nor can they provide chemotherapy or other ongoing treatments. The team should, however, assess any patient who presents and manage any immediately treatable conditions, including pain and infection. Appropriate advice may be offered along with referral to an appropriate facility.

Rehabilitation[8]

Rehabilitation is an essential component of an emergency medical team. This will ensure the best recovery from injury but also, and most importantly, facilitate the rapid and safe discharge of patients, thereby increasing capacity for new admissions. Rehabilitation teams can also deploy as a specialised facility to 'bolt on' to another team or embed within a MoH facility.

The WHO World report on disability defines rehabilitation as "a set of measures that assist individuals who experience, or are likely to experience, disability to achieve and maintain optimal functioning in interaction with their environments".

Rehabilitation professionals who are integrated into EMTs in the acute phase of a response are likely to see people with a broad range of injuries and conditions and should therefore be adequately experienced in trauma and medical rehabilitation. Specialised rehabilitation skills become increasingly necessary as patients with amputations and spinal cord injuries progress or gaps in clinical specialisation are identified; the EMT should therefore plan the inclusion of appropriately qualified professionals to meet this need after the acute phase of care.

Rehabilitation professionals with an arriving team should be experienced in trauma and medical rehabilitation with experience and/or training to work in austere environments. They should comply with the same requirements for practice as in their home country (such as professional registration and licensing) and should work within their scope of practice. Those from countries in which there is no professional certification may practice under the direction and authority of their EMT clinical lead with approval of the ministry of health of the host country.

Type 1 EMTs should be able to provide basic rehabilitation care or refer patients to an appropriate EMT or existing local facility. Type 2 and 3 EMTs, with one or more rehabilitation professionals, should be able to autonomously provide rehabilitation for patients (including paediatric and geriatric patients) with:

- fractures, including those with external fixation or traction;
- amputation; peripheral nerve injury;
- burns, grafts, or flaps.

Type 2 and 3 EMTs should be able to provide early rehabilitation to patients with acquired brain injury and spinal cord injury while they await specialist rehabilitation. The essential clinical rehabilitation skills to be represented in the EMT are listed in Table 9.5.

Rehabilitation professionals should be deployed primarily on the basis of their demonstrated essential skills; however, those deployed within the first 2 weeks of response should have at least 2 years of clinical experience, and more if working in a

Table 9.5 Essential Clinical Rehabilitation Skills

- basic splinting
- assistive device prescription fitting and training
- positioning and patient mobilisation, including early mobilisation
- education and re-training of patients and care providers in daily activities
- provision of psycho-social support, for example, psychological first aid
- respiratory care, including sputum clearance techniques

specialisation. EMTs are encouraged to prepare terms of reference for rehabilitation professionals and define team roles before deployment. Rotation of rehabilitation staff will be decided by the EMT; however, a minimum stay of 3 weeks is recommended to provide continuity of care, with sufficient time being planned for handover. Efforts should be made to maintain consistency in the treatment approaches of different rehabilitation professionals by the use of guidelines, protocols, and common pre-deployment training.

DEALING WITH THE DEAD[9]

When responding to disasters, including conflicts, it is almost inevitable that at some point there will be a large number of unburied dead. This is very distressing; the smell is overwhelming, and their presence provokes the fear of epidemics amongst survivors. This fear is not unreasonable but is unfounded, and not supported by the evidence. At its worst, this fear leads to precipitous burial and mass graves, with terrible long-term consequences for families in establishing whether their loved ones have in fact died, and if so, where their bodies might lie. Mass graves should, therefore, be avoided if at all possible.

In a sudden-onset disaster (rather than a disease outbreak), the unburied dead pose little or no threat to the living. If there is to be a spontaneous disease outbreak, it will be from the mass movement of the living into inadequate living conditions with its consequent poor water quality, sanitation, and hygiene, leading to increased cases of infectious and diarrhoeal disease. Of course, if death is from an infectious disease that survives after the death of its host, then there is a risk. However, in practice this is essentially limited to the viral haemorrhagic fevers (for example, Ebola) and cholera. It is to be noted that cholera is not an inevitable consequence of a sudden-onset disaster. Inadequate WASH can facilitate its transmission, but usually only when and where it is already endemic. However, the cholera epidemic that followed the earthquake in Haiti, where it was not endemic, came some months afterwards, and is now recognised as having been brought into the country by international workers.

The profound haemolysis that accompanies the end stages of diseases such as Ebola leads to bleeding and leakage of serous fluid from bodily orifices, making the handling of the body after death a high-risk operation. The washing of the body by family members is a cultural practice across many countries, and certainly during the outbreak of Ebola in West Africa, it led to widespread transmission of a disease which could potentially be contained due to its lack of aerosol spread. It is essential that those handling the bodies of those who have died from cholera and any viral haemorrhagic fever wear full *personal protection equipment* (PPE) and the body be sealed within a fully enclosed body bag.

Bodies will, of course, decompose, but this process, though unpleasant to witness and perhaps even more unpleasant to smell, does not of itself cause or transmit disease. Bodies obviously contain faeces, but these are largely contained within the body itself. There may be some leakage as the anal sphincter relaxes, but again this will be confined to the immediate area around the body. Only if a person handling the body is contaminated by effluent and touches their mouth will infection be possible, and then only in creating an individual case of a diarrhoeal disease. It will not cause an epidemic. Dead bodies have not been shown to contaminate the water table.

> After a sudden-onset disaster, even large numbers of unburied dead bodies pose little or no threat to the physical health of survivors or rescuers.

NOTES AND REFERENCES

1. https://www.rcsed.ac.uk/events-courses
2. https://www.rcseng.ac.uk/education-and-exams/courses
3. ICRC. War Surgery—Working with Limited Resources in Armed Conflict and Other Situations of Violence Volume 1. International Committee of the Red Cross; 2022. https://www.icrc.org/en/publication/0973-war-surgery-working-limited-resources-armed-conflict-and-other-situations-violence
4. https://resources.relabhs.org//resource/management-of-limb-injuries-during-disasters-and-conflicts/
5. http://www.who.int/mental_health/publications/guide_field_workers/en/
6. www.who.int/entity/mental_health/emergencies/facilitator_manual_2014/en/
7. https://www.diabetes.co.uk/diabetes-medication/gluca-gon-injection-kit.html
8. https://www.who.int/publications/i/item/emergency-medical-teams
9. PAHO/WHO. Management of Dead Bodies after Disasters: A Field Manual for First Responders. 2nd edition (Revised)—PAHO/WHO (Pan American Health Organization); 2018. https://www.paho.org/en/documents/management-dead-bodies-after-disasters-field-manual-first-responders-2nd-edition-revised

10

Infectious Diseases and Outbreak Response

A field hospital must have the capacity to establish a separate tent as a designated isolation area. The tent should be well ventilated with fresh air and with a 2-metre gap between beds. It must be clearly marked, and patients must have access to separate toilet and handwashing facilities. This isolation tent should not be a medium- to long-term solution, but rather a short-term measure as referral and transfer of these patients to a specialist isolation and treatment is prioritised.

Four major communicable diseases account for the majority of deaths in humanitarian emergencies. These are:

- diarrhoeal diseases
- respiratory infections
- measles
- malaria

The need for EMTs to respond to surgical health emergencies such as earthquakes is becoming outweighed by the increasing demand for medical support for disease outbreaks. The WHO global surveillance system continuously monitors threats to public health and, when necessary, will activate the Global Outbreak Alert and Response Network (GOARN). The EMT initiative is an important component of the global response, with teams responding to

 DOI: 10.1201/9781003473718-10

disease outbreaks including COVID-19, diphtheria, measles, and Ebola in recent years. As well as providing additional healthcare professionals to strengthen the response network, EMTs can also provide technical support and training when requested. Teams that respond are required to have been fully trained in safe working practices in the presence of dangerous pathogens and have in place robust protocols for the safe donning and doffing of PPE.

Teams that deploy must have a dedicated *infection prevention and control* (IPC) lead. The IPC lead will be responsible for the training and monitoring in PPE donning and doffing. They will set up a donning and doffing area near the isolation area close to a handwashing facility. Doffing of PPE should be done in an order that minimises cross-contamination and under the supervision of the IPC lead or a designated colleague. PPE includes gloves, apron or isolation gown, eye protection, and face mask (surgical) or respirator (FFP3).

The viral haemorrhagic fevers, Ebola in particular, probably command the most public attention, but cholera remains one of the most frequent and deadliest, and tragically one of the most preventable, infectious diseases. Malaria also remains a major killer, particularly of children, and is preventable. The principal preventative measures involve draining stagnant water and vector control.

STAGNANT WATER DRAINAGE

All stagnant water should be drained, including water storage containers and other water accumulation sites, such as abandoned plastic cups, used tyres, broken bottles, and flowerpots.

VECTOR CONTROL

Indoor residual spraying (IRS)[1] with an insecticide is an important vector (mosquito) control measure, but should cover 80% of dwellings in order to be effective. Distribution of *long-lasting insecticidal nets* (LLINs)[2] (guided by entomological assessment and expertise) is also useful. The priority in distribution is to hospital patients, severely malnourished people, pregnant women, and children less than 2 years old. The distribution of untreated nets is not recommended.

It is imperative that team members adhere to their team's malaria prophylaxis guidelines, tailored to the country of deployment.[3] The team must also have guidelines in place for the treatment of malaria, again adapted to location, the type of malaria, and the presence of resistant strains.

Teams must have in their laboratory a rapid test for malaria and begin treatment for *P. Falciparum* malaria immediately on diagnosis. In most parts of the world, *P. Falciparum* is now resistant to chloroquine, and artemisinin combination therapy is used. Detailed guidelines are available for malaria treatment.[4]

Cholera

Cholera is an acute diarrhoeal disease that can kill within hours if left untreated. It is a disease of poverty, affecting people with inadequate access to safe water and basic sanitation; conflict, unplanned urbanisation, and climate change all increase the risk of a disease outbreak. It has been estimated that each year there are 1.3 to 4.0 million cases of cholera, and 21,000 to 143,000 deaths worldwide.

Most people infected with cholera have no, or only mild, symptoms and can be successfully treated with oral rehydration solution. Severe cases will need rapid treatment with intravenous fluids and antibiotics. Provision of safe water, basic sanitation, and promotion of safe hygiene practices are critical to preventing and controlling the transmission of cholera and other waterborne diseases. Oral cholera vaccines should be used in conjunction with improvements in water and sanitation for the control of cholera outbreaks and for prevention in areas known to be at high risk. A global strategy on cholera control, *Ending cholera: a global roadmap to 2030*, with a target to reduce cholera deaths by 90%, was launched in 2017. The causes and treatment of cholera are covered comprehensively in publications produced by the WHO.[5]

Other Diarrhoeal Illnesses

There are other causes of acute watery diarrhoea.[6] Among children under 5 years of age, the most common viral pathogens are rotavirus, norovirus, adenovirus, and astrovirus. Potential bacterial pathogens include *Escherichia coli, Salmonella spp.*(species/subspecies),

Shigella spp., and Campylobacter spp., while parasitic pathogens include *Cryptosporidium, Giardia*, and *Entamoeba spp.* Rotavirus and *E. coli* are the most common pathogens among children across all age groups, while parasitic pathogens are prevalent in children aged 3–5 years. Bacterial pathogens, including *E. coli, Salmonella*, and *Shigella*, are common in children in the 6- to 10-year age group, as are rotavirus, norovirus, and sapovirus. Location-specific etiologic patterns also need to be considered (WHO data).

PREVENTION OF DIARRHOEAL DISEASE

The primary prevention of diarrhoeal disease is to stop water from becoming contaminated with human faeces, for example from sewage, septic tanks, and latrines. Animal faeces also contain micro-organisms which, if allowed to contaminate water sources, can cause diarrhoea. The causative organisms of diarrhoeal disease can also spread from person to person; this will clearly be aggravated by poor personal hygiene.

Food which is undercooked or prepared or stored in unhygienic conditions is another major cause of diarrhoea, as is unsafe domestic water storage and handling. Fish and seafood from polluted water may also contribute to the outbreak of disease. Key measures to prevent diarrhoea are shown in Table 10.1.

Treatment of diarrhoea includes rehydration with oral rehydration salts (ORS) solution. ORS is a mixture of clean water, salt, and sugar. It costs a few cents/pence per treatment. ORS is absorbed in the small intestine and replaces the water and electrolytes lost in faeces. Zinc supplements reduce the duration of a diarrhoeal

Table 10.1 Key Measures in Preventing (Non-Cholera) Diarrhoeal Illness

- access to safe drinking-water
- use of improved sanitation
- hand washing with soap
- exclusive breastfeeding for the first 6 months of life
- good personal and food hygiene
- health education about how infections spread
- rotavirus vaccination.

episode by 25% and are associated with a 30% reduction in stool volume. Rehydration with intravenous fluids may be necessary in cases of severe dehydration or shock. The vicious circle of malnutrition and diarrhoea can be broken by continuing to give nutrient-rich foods—including breast milk—during an episode, and by providing a nutritious diet—including exclusive breastfeeding for the first 6 months of life—to children when they are well. A health professional may sometimes be needed, particularly for the management of persistent diarrhoea or when there is blood in the stool or signs of dehydration.

Clinically, diarrhoea can be divided into

- acute watery diarrhoea—lasts several hours or days and includes cholera
- acute bloody diarrhoea—also called dysentery

Dysentery is highly infectious and is passed on hand-to-mouth. Patients have abdominal pain, nausea and vomiting, and a high temperature. Shigella is the commonest infective agent.

Salmonella is a common cause of food poisoning leading to diarrhoea. However, Salmonella typhi produces typhoid fever. This causes fever, abdominal pain, and a range of symptoms including headache and vomiting. A characteristic red rash—rose-coloured spots—may develop. Typhoid fever is spread by the faecal-oral route. Treatment is with antibiotics.

AMOEBIC DYSENTERY

Amoebiasis is caused by the parasite *Entamoeba histolytica*. Diagnosis is aided by its known prevalence in an area and by stool microscopy (Figure 10.1). There are also specific antigen/antibody tests. If left untreated, the infection may spread from the intestine to the liver where abscesses can form. In rare circumstances, there is further dissemination and brain abscess may occur. Fulminant amoebiasis, presenting as peritonitis due to intestinal perforation, is a rare but life-threatening complication. Standard treatment is with metronidazole plus a luminal agent (paromomycin and diloxanide furoate).[7]

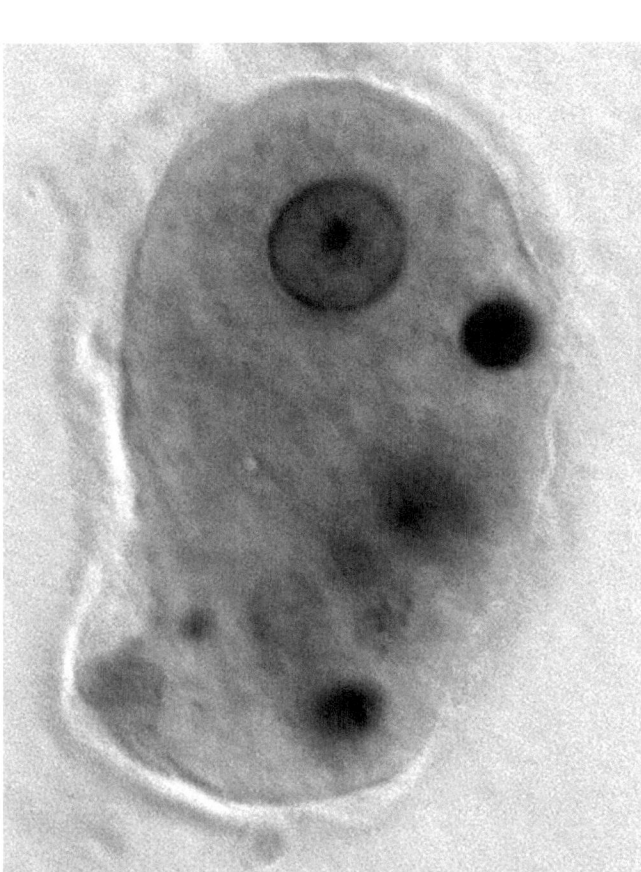

Figure 10.1 *Entamoeba histolytica*

USE OF DRUGS FOR CHILDREN WITH DIARRHOEA

Antibiotics should only be used for dysentery and for suspected cholera cases with severe dehydration. Otherwise, they are ineffective and should not be given. Antidiarrhoeal drugs and antiemetics have no proven value and can be dangerous.

Women and Children

Pregnancy and childbirth are normal phenomena in any community, and babies continue to be born despite situations of conflict and catastrophe. It is estimated that 1 in 5 of all women of childbearing age within a population will be pregnant at any one time. Consequently, every deploying team must expect to look after pregnant and labouring women, and to provide standard neonatal care, including basic life support as required. Globally, 75% of maternal deaths are due to 5 causes, namely:

- haemorrhage
- sepsis
- obstructed labour
- eclampsia/severe pre-eclampsia
- miscarriage/abortion.

All emergency medical teams must be able to provide basic emergency obstetric care (EmOC). This includes administration of parenteral antibiotics, uterotonic drugs, and magnesium sulphate for pre-eclampsia and eclampsia, assisted vaginal delivery (forceps and ventouse), manual removal of placenta, removal of retained products of conception (by manual vacuum aspiration or curettage), and care of the newborn, including basic neonatal resuscitation.

In principle, a Type 1 EMT deployment provides basic EmOC, whereas a Type 2 EMT deployment provides comprehensive EmOC, including caesarean section. 'Newborn' and 'neonatal' are terms that refer to the first 28 days of life. The mortality risk during the neonatal period is highest at the time of birth and decreases over the subsequent days and weeks. Up to 36% of neonatal deaths occur within the first 24 hours of birth and nearly 73% in the first week of life. Worldwide, 44% of deaths in children younger than 5 years now occur in the first month of life. Around 5% of infants do not take their first breath spontaneously. Almost all of these babies respond well to bag-valve-mask ventilation. With lung inflation, there is a rapid rise in heart rate, which is assessed by auscultation.

Children are especially vulnerable to increased rates of morbidity and mortality in a disaster due to a greater risk of communicable and vector-borne diseases, which is compounded by poorer baseline health, incomplete immunisation schedules, and malnutrition.[8]

NOTES AND REFERENCES

1. https://www.who.int/publications
2. https://www.who.int/news/item/16-11-2016-five-year-who-investigation-shows-that-llins-remain-a-highly-effective-tool-in-the-malaria-fightt
3. https://assets.publishing.service.gov.uk
4. https://bnf.nice.org.uk/treatment-summaries
5. https://www.who.int/news-room/fact-sheets/detail/cholera
6. https://www.who.int/news-room/fact-sheets/detail/diarrhoeal-disease
7. Amoebiasis—Symptoms, Diagnosis and Treatment. *BMJ Best Practice.* https://bestpractice.bmj.com/topics/en-gb/553
8. World Health Organization. Manual for the Health Care of Children in Humanitarian Emergencies. Geneva: WHO; 2008.

11

Triage

The word 'triage' originates from the French word *trier,* meaning to sort. Baron Larrey introduced the concept into Napoleon's army where patients were sorted (triaged) into categories of urgency based on their clinical condition and not their military rank.

Triage decisions in humanitarian emergencies can be:

- to do the most for the most
- to treat the sickest first, or the most likely to survive
- to alter the level of care provided to an individual in order to maintain the highest standard of care to the population

It is important to understand that triage requires getting senior, experienced people up to the front, and that it is not a one-off event but is continuous and dynamic (Figure 11.1).

MASS CASUALTY MANAGEMENT

The *SIEVE* triage tool can be used to determine a patient's priority (Figure 11.2). There are 4 categories. The most urgent are those whose life is obviously in immediate danger and require **immediate** treatment (**priority 1**). These patients usually have airways obstruction or catastrophic haemorrhage.

Next are patients whose lives are not in immediate danger but who will require a surgical or medical intervention **within**

DOI: 10.1201/9781003473718-11

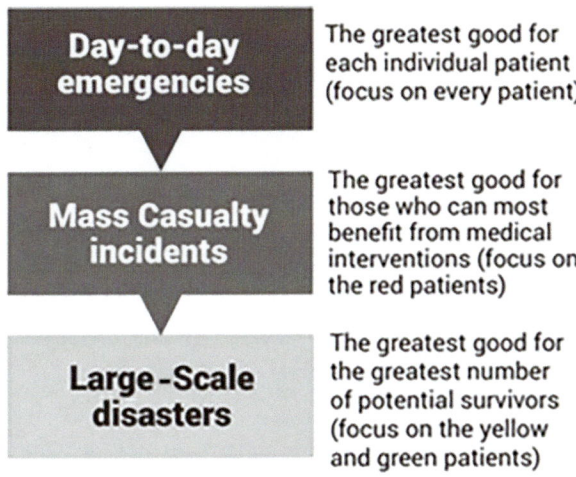

Figure 11.1 Different approaches to triage

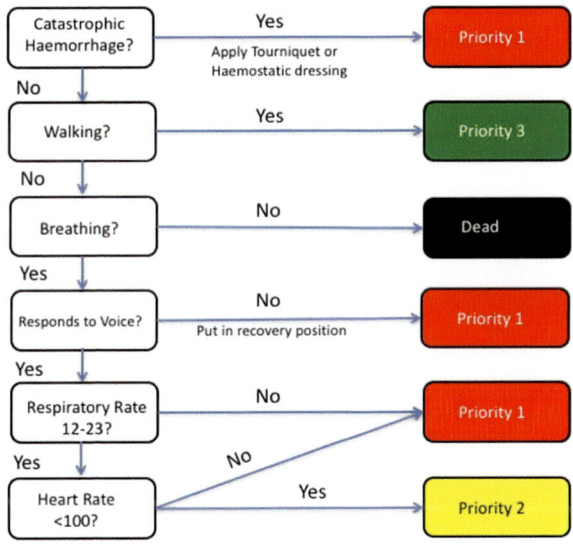

Figure 11.2 The triage sieve

2 to 4 hours (**priority 2**), for example, intra-abdominal bleeding or complicated fractures. The next group consists of those with minor injuries who will require treatment at some point but not immediately and are therefore **delayed (priority 3)**. Minor fractures or lacerations are commonly placed in this group.

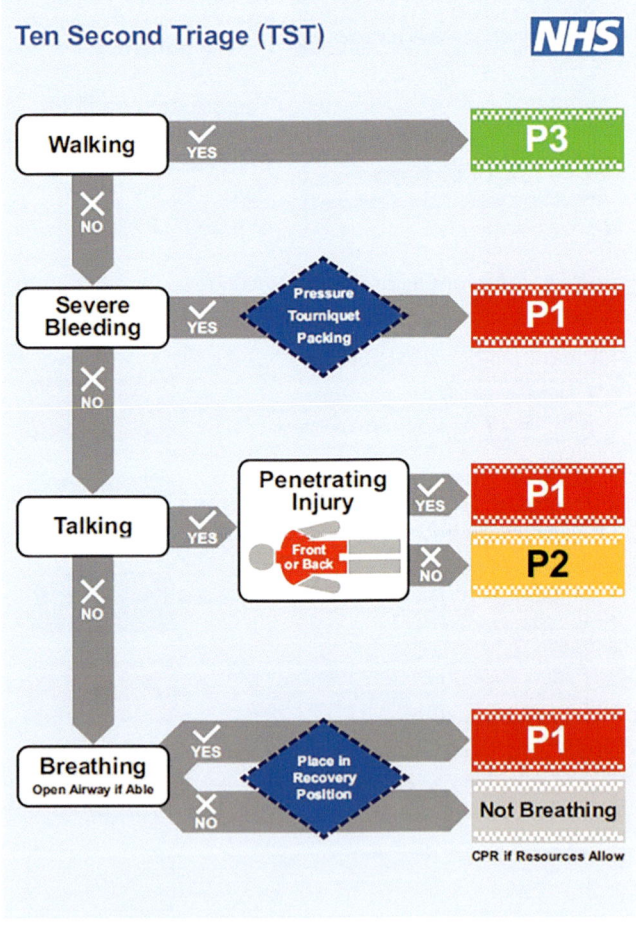

Figure 11.3 Ten-second triage

The final group can be the most difficult group to manage, that is, those whose injuries are obviously so extensive that they cannot be saved with the resources available. This **'expectant'** category can raise ethical issues within the team and provoke strong emotional reactions. These should have been addressed prior to deployment and during training, but they can still arise during deployment and must be addressed during debriefing after the incident.

The triage sieve follows a defined series of steps beginning with an assessment of the presence or absence of catastrophic haemorrhage. If there is life-threatening severe haemorrhage, the patient is automatically a PRIORITY 1. If there is no such bleeding and the patient *can* walk (not *is walking*), the category is PRIORITY 3. If the patient is not able to walk, a breathing assessment is carried out: if the casualty is not breathing, they are DEAD. If they are breathing but do not respond to voice, they should be put in the recovery position and labelled PRIORITY 1. If they respond to voice and a respiratory rate check is outside the range of 12–23, they are also PRIORITY 1. If the respiratory rate is between 12 and 23 and on checking their pulse it is <100, they are PRIORITY 2. If the pulse is above 100, they are PRIORITY 1.

There is currently a great deal of active research ongoing into effective reproduceable triage methods, and the traditional triage SORT is now rarely used due to intra-user variability and difficulty and delay in completing it. "Ten-second triage" offers another potential method of emergency triage for large numbers of casualties (Figure 11.3).

Whichever method of triage is chosen, it must be reproducible, consistant when applied by different clinicians, and simple and straightforward to use.

12

Working in Another Country

CULTURAL ISSUES

Responding to humanitarian emergencies carries with it a number of ethical dilemmas to which there are often no hard and fast answers but for which team members must be prepared. No matter how well resourced the team, the scale of the emergency may be such that care that might be given in other circumstances cannot be provided or must even be withheld. Decisions regarding when to treat or when not to treat are amongst the most difficult. The burden of decision-making need not fall on the shoulders of one person. Teams should have identified before deployment an emergency ethical committee amongst their numbers to which team members can refer such difficult decisions and receive a rapid consensus view. It is important that the team understands such collective responsibility.

Attention must be paid to local culture and customs, but this can bring about conflict when local custom and practice may be at odds with the team's own medical standards. This may be manifest, for example, in the priority of care given to men over women, the level of confidentiality afforded to women patients, and equity of care across social or ethnic groups. Issues such as women being examined only by women must be accommodated as far as

 DOI: 10.1201/9781003473718-12

possible as one would in one's home country, although in emergencies this may be difficult to achieve at all times. The differing treatment of men and women in society needs to be understood and accepted if it does not prejudice the safe treatment of patients.

Nevertheless, teams should try their best to accommodate local custom and practice, and where this appears to be at significant odds with their own ethical values, they should consult both as a team and more broadly with the WHO and local authorities. Some of these issues are addressed on the Royal College of Surgeons of Edinburgh's *Introduction to Humanitarian Healthcare* online course.

It is essential that incoming teams gain acceptance by the host community, as this is an important way of staying safe and gaining local information. The community needs to understand why the team is there, what it is doing, why it is doing it, and that it is working with the local community. It is important to be respectful of local social and religious customs, whether one necessarily agrees with them or not, and even if it makes one sometimes feel uncomfortable; an example might be head coverings for female staff in Muslim communities.

All patients have a right to privacy, and humanitarian emergencies are not an exception. Organisations look to use imagery to promote their work, but if patients are involved the same rules of confidentiality and permission apply as they do in the UK. It is important that any consent, to photography for example, is truly informed and not inadvertently understood to be a condition of treatment.

SECURITY

Working to ensure that one is welcome within a community does not mean that one doesn't need to take appropriate measures to keep safe. Basic measures include curfews for staff after dark, avoiding certain areas of a town or village, always using designated drivers, and ensuring that team members never travel alone. Rigid communication protocols must be in place in order to ensure that the team leader knows where its members are at all times. It must be made clear in the 'rules of engagement' that it is the responsibility of each individual team member to ensure that they are familiar with the security plan. Regular security briefings should be held, and team members encouraged to discuss and raise any issues or concerns. Ultimately, however, there must be an individual—the team leader or head of organisation—who will make the final decisions concerning security, and these decisions need to be followed rigorously for the safety of all.

There are occasional missions into conflicts when armed guards and armed escorts whilst travelling are necessary to protect a team in an extreme situation. Any decision to implement these measures will be taken at a senior level, and not locally. Factored into the decision-making process will be how using armed guards will be viewed by the local community and whether having such guards will increase rather than reduce vulnerability. Ultimately, if protection is thought to be required, the question arises as to whether or not the team should be deployed to that location. The use of armed guards and/or the military to provide this protection must align with the humanitarian principles. It is worth noting that the risks for international staff may be different to the risks for local staff, and sometimes it is possible that programmes can be delivered more safely by national or local staff alone.

Security can be divisive when there are different rules for national and international staff. International staff in a field hospital may be evacuated if the situation deteriorates, whilst national colleagues may not. Similarly, national staff recruited into the team may be able to work night shifts, but international staff may not be due to security concerns. Being aware of these differences and the impact on national staff is key to teams working well together.

In summary, to keep a team and their patients safe, it is important to undertake an effective security assessment, put in place strong security measures, continually update the security assessment, and communicate this information regularly to the team members.

MEDEVAC

As we have said, the members of teams that deploy to humanitarian emergencies must have comprehensive travel and health insurance that includes medical evacuation and repatriation. The majority of policies are likely to require initial evacuation to the nearest suitable facility in the case of an emergency, and then repatriation home when stable.

A recurring pressure for teams is the demand from patients, their relatives, the media, and sometimes local officials or politicians for patients to be transferred to another, better resourced country, usually one's own. The pressure to do this must not be underestimated—a pressure that may not just be from outside of the team, but also from among its members. However well-intentioned, such requests are never straightforward and are fraught with moral and legal issues if shortcuts are taken and international protocols and laws are not followed.

If requests are made for treatment in another country, the authorities in that country will have to approve their immigration and issue appropriate travel documents. This process is usually government to government. An approach to the relevant MoH may start the process, which will then be carried out through formal channels. In many humanitarian crises, the UN will establish a medevac committee on which will sit representatives of the local ministry of health, the UN, and the WHO. Medevac committees are important because the demand for transfer to another country will usually exceed the availability of places, and a triage system will need to be established. Sometimes the approach is to list certain types of conditions which are eligible, for example, eminently treatable conditions without long-term complications, and conditions that are ineligible, particularly chronic, incurable, and terminal conditions. A more flexible approach is to have no exclusion criteria but instead place patients in order of priority so that rather than be permanently excluded, patients may gain inclusion when there is no one with greater priority.

The medical evacuation of children can be particularly complex. A child will usually not be evacuated by themselves but at the very least must travel with one parent. Of course, parents do not want to be separated from their child, nor from each other or their other children, so in practical terms, the evacuation of one child may mean the evacuation of a family. If treatment in the host country is prolonged and the patient and/or their siblings get embedded in the school system, then later repatriation becomes more complicated.

Special consideration must be given to orphaned or 'abandoned' babies and children. In the aftermath of a humanitarian crisis, children may be separated from their parents and appear to have been abandoned or left alone in hospital. While this may be the case, the assumption must never be made in haste, and every effort must be made to contact the parents or relatives. UNICEF, which has a special responsibility in this regard, must be consulted and will liaise with the local authorities. It is essential that it is never assumed that a child is truly orphaned or has been abandoned until at least 3 months have passed.

Summary

Humanitarian medicine is complex, often difficult, but can be very rewarding. It is, however, important to recognise that like any other field of medical practice, it requires training, experience, and appropriate qualifications.

There are national and international structures, as described in this book, that are available for the coordination of international emergency responses and matching their capabilities to the needs they have identified. Foremost among these is the Emergency Medical Teams Initiative at WHO, a full knowledge of which is essential for anyone who wishes to work in the humanitarian sector.

Given the developments in the organisation and structure of the international emergency medical response there is no place now for inexperienced individuals to respond uninvited. The potential for doing more harm than good is too great.

Humanitarian work brings many rewards and I encourage the reader to consider deployment. It also carries emotional and ethical pressures, the effects of which though can be mitigated by adequate preparation and training, and only deploying with an experienced, well established, and well-resourced organisation.

If you are interested, do consider the following.

First complete your full training in whatever is your background specialty/discipline and attend additional specialist humanitarian skills courses.

During or after your clinical training, consider gaining additional qualifications such as a Masters degree in public health, disaster management, humanitarian and conflict studies etc. These are very valuable in expanding your understanding of how humanitarian emergencies arise and evolve.

In addition, explore clinical courses leading to diplomas, for example in the UK there is "Medicine in Conflict and Catastrophe" at the Society of Apothecaries, or Tropical Medicine at the London/Liverpool Schools. These provide further opportunities to expand both knowledge and skill base.

Finally join the humanitarian community. Most large NGOs will have their support groups, volunteers, and fundraisers. At many universities they will have their own student groups. An important development in the humanitarian community has been the establishment of a "professional home" in the Faculty of Remote Rural and Humanitarian Healthcare at the Royal College of Surgeons of Edinburgh. This is open to all those involved in this work and from anywhere in the world.

Index

Note: **Boldface** page references indicate tables. *Italic* references indicate figures and boxed text.